Risk Factors for Cardiovascular Disease in Non-Smokers

International Workshop, Washington, Tyne and Wear, May 11, 1991

# Risk Factors for Cardiovascular Disease in Non-Smokers

Editors
*Donald F. Weetman*, Sunderland
*Diana Wood*, Bradford

12 figures and 21 tables, 1993



KARGER

Basel · Freiburg · Paris · London · New York · New Delhi · Bangkok · Singapore · Tokyo · Sydney

Library of Congress Cataloging-in-Publication Data
International Workshop on Risk Factors for Cardiovascular Disease in Non-smokers
(1991: Washington, Tyne and Wear, England)
Risk factors for cardiovascular disease in non-smokers / editors, Donald F. Weetman, Diana Wood.
Includes bibliographical references and index.
1. Cardiovascular system – Diseases – Risk factors – Congresses.
I. Weetman, Donald F. II. Wood, Diana. III. Title.
RA645.C34I587 1991
616.1'071 – dc20
ISBN 3-8055-5682-9

Drug Dosage
The authors and the publisher have exerted every effort to ensure that drug selection and dosage set forth in this text are in accord with current recommendations and practice at the time of publication. However, in view of ongoing research, changes in government regulations, and the constant flow of information relating to drug therapy and drug reactions, the reader is urged to check the package insert for each drug for any change in indications and dosage and for added warnings and precautions. This is particularly important when the recommended agent is a new and/or infrequently employed drug.


Printed in Switzerland on acid-free paper by Thür AG Offsetdruck, Pratteln
ISBN 3-8055-5682-9

# Contents

# Preface

In recent years, there have been substantial changes in education at the first-degree level in the United Kingdom. Many institutions have changed their status from that of the former Polytechnics to Universities; many new courses have been designed, and modern teaching techniques introduced. From the inevitable commotion surrounding these developments, a new and exciting challenge has confronted the professional educators.

Amongst the subjects that are now being read at degree level by some students at Sunderland, for example, is a new course in Health Sciences. At least one of the intended career destinations from this degree is a position in health education, whereby the nonspecialist will receive advice on a healthy lifestyle from our graduates. The modern techniques of education that are being employed include a new emphasis on the processes by which students learn, this sometimes sheltering under the new key phrase 'student-centred learning'. These changes have required much re-evaluation of the existing working practices.

In this context, it seemed worthwhile to attempt to collect together in one place much of the relevant source material on cardiovascular disease. It is generally accepted that cardiovascular disease is the leading cause of death, particularly premature death, in virtually every culture. The age-standardized annual mortality rate for males between the ages of 35 and 64 years varies about 15-fold country by country (from around 30/100,000 in Japan to 450/100,000 in North Karelia, Finland [1]). In all countries, the rates are lower for females than males. There is a vast literature about why these differences occur from country to country and from men to women, but what do we really know? This question was one of the starting points of the workshop. It also seemed worthwhile to attempt the new approach of considering non-smokers, because these are in the majority in virtually all societies.

High quality education can be achieved only if there is due attention paid to the reliability of data obtained from different investigative techniques. Furthermore, a consideration of numbers in an abstract manner seems flawed, unless there is regard to the possible mechanisms by which death results. It was within this set of assumptions that the workshop was planned.

It was possible to contact and make arrangements with the distinguished team of speakers only with the very considerable help of the organizing committee: Dr. A.J.S. Gardiner (Airdrie), Prof. A.R. Lorimer (Glasgow), G.B. Leslie Esq. (Biggleswade) and Dr. J. Munby (Sunderland). I am very grateful for the expert advice and help of this committee.

My deepest thanks are due to many individuals who helped the workshop to run smoothly. It seems that little can be achieved in an academic department without the help of the chief technician: I am most grateful to our own excellent chief, Norman Turner, for sorting out all those apparently little difficulties, which make the difference between a crisis and a well-organized event. The text of the present book was arrived at by several processes, not least of which was from a very accurate transcription of the presentations and discussions made expertly by Carol-Ann Lyme. Finally, and perhaps most of all for organizing the smooth running of the workshop, I am deeply indebted to the totally unflappable Julie C. Fleming, the Business Development Manager of the Washington Conference Centre: I can wholeheartedly recommend the organizational skills of Ms. Fleming and the University facilities at Washington to any prospective workshop, conference or small course convenor.

I would like to express thanks to my co-editor, Dr. Diana Wood, for her patience, skill and persistence in bringing the manuscripts and transcriptions to an accurate and readable state. It seems that I have not contributed that much to the present volume, but, of course, any errors and omissions are entirely my responsibility.

It has been a pleasure to work with the splendid team of specialists in medical publishing at S. Karger AG, Basel, Switzerland, without whose help the workshop would not have been published.

Prof. *D.F. Weetman*

School of Health Sciences,
University of Sunderland

## *Reference*

1 Karvonen MJ: Health challenges of the developed world. Hygie 1992;11, Suppl:18–23.

# Welcome Address

It is my pleasure to welcome you to this workshop on Risk Factors for Cardiovascular Diseases in Non-Smokers.

It is not only welcome to the University of Sunderland, but welcome to the University of Sunderland at Washington. The University has around 8,000 students, reading a broad range of subjects that range from art and design through business, humanities, social studies, education, life sciences, health sciences, physical sciences, maths, computing and engineering. One achievement of which we are particularly proud is that the sandwich-course idea originated early in this century, when the Institution was a Technical College. One of the better known features of the University of Sunderland at the moment is that it is very well regarded in the field of pharmaceutical sciences, pharmacy, pharmacology etc., and in fact has the broadest and biggest range of educational provision in this subject area of any institution in the United Kingdom.

We have an increasing interest in the health sciences, and that is one of the reasons for arranging this workshop. Why non-smokers? I have been led to understand that the organizing committee adopted this title because so much has been said and written about the effects of smoking on health. Perhaps a new approach will reveal new truths, but we will not be able to decide this until the end of a very busy day. We all have much to consider.

*J.R. Brown*

Dean of the Faculty of Science,
University of Sunderland, UK

# Preamble and Context

Weetman DF, Wood D (eds): Risk Factors for Cardiovascular Disease in Non-Smokers.
Int. Workshop, Washington, Tyne and Wear, 1991. Basel, Karger, 1993, pp 1–6

## Risk Factors for Cardiovascular Disease in Non-Smokers: An Overview

*A.C. Rankin, M. Mandawat, A.R. Lorimer*
Royal Infirmary, Glasgow, UK

There is general agreement as to the importance of vascular disease and its impact on the community. Why should this be so? A historical perspective is justified. The Royal Infirmary of Glasgow, the Institute in which we work, was founded in 1792. The community recognized the need for a hospital to deal with the clamant clinical problems of the time. These were mainly infectious diseases, including cholera. When the Infirmary was rebuilt in the early years of this century, Glasgow had become a teeming industrial city and the clinical problems were those associated with an environment of pollution and overcrowding – tuberculosis, rickets and respiratory disease. Time moves on and the clinical emphasis has again changed. We are now required to investigate and manage diseases that have come to the forefront as others have been controlled. Foremost among these is atherosclerosis and its protean consequences involving diverse tissues and organs. There is a progressive narrowing of the arterial lumen, a progressive reduction in blood supply and potential for vascular catastrophe in, for example, brain, heart and limbs.

The aetiology of atherosclerosis has been debated, often fiercely, for many years. Rokitansky, around 1842, suggested that the initial event was likely to be thrombus and that the deposit on the arterial wall was due to the subsequent degeneration of the thrombus. Virchow however had a contrary view, believing that the degenerative process began in the arterial wall and that thrombus was a later, superadded effect. We now believe that both are important.

A generally accepted theory at present links together narrowing of the arterial wall due to the accumulation of lipid with the development of thrombus due to interaction between the atherosclerotic plaque and formed elements of the blood, particularly platelets. The arterial lining, the endothelium, is of considerable importance. The response to injury hypothesis [1] states that repeated injury to the endothelium will lead to proliferation of connective tissue components, to lipoprotein accumulation and to the development of a lipid-rich plaque. The centre of the plaque may rupture and cause platelet aggregation. This aggregation of platelets is due to the release of chemotaxic compounds, including prostaglandins. Free radicals might also be relevant in this situation. Accumulation of platelets can initiate a coagulation cascade leading to the accumulation of thrombus on the damaged endothelium. In addition, platelets release platelet-derived growth factor (PDGF) which encourages migration of smooth muscle cells into the area. The 'mature' atherosclerotic plaque will contain lipoprotein components, collagen deposits, smooth muscle cells that have migrated from the media of the arterial wall and has the potential for plaque ulceration and rupture to initiate a major thrombotic vascular occlusion.

Cardiovascular disease presents a major health problem. It is responsible for 50% of the deaths of men aged 45–54 years. The mortality varies from country to country with levels in Scotland and Finland being currently among the highest in the world [2]. Within the United Kingdom there are striking regional variations with the risk increasing from the south-east to the north. There is no need to regard the high death rate from coronary disease in the United Kingdom as being inevitable. In the United States, Canada and Australia there has been a fall of up to 20% [3]. Epidemiology allows us to study disease in communities rather than in individuals. Certain characteristics in apparently healthy persons have subsequently been shown to be related to the development of coronary and other vascular diseases. It must be emphasized that the concept of 'risk factors' does not imply a causal role in atherosclerotic disease. The fact of an association does not imply a cause. They are merely indicators of risk. When recognized as such the study of risk factors has provided much valuable information. Coronary risk factors have to be considered and reconsidered in order to arrive at a coherent, practical and balanced strategy for the prevention and management of coronary heart disease (CHD).

This review deals with risk factors in non-smokers. The role of cigarette smoking, both active and passive, will therefore not be considered further. It should however be emphasized that cigarette smoking is probably the most important risk factor for CHD with a rate in smokers of 2–3 times that of non-smokers [4, 5]. This review is not intended to be exhaustive but seek to emphasize areas of recent advance.

### *Plasma Cholesterol*

The importance of plasma cholesterol as a risk is well known. The Seven Countries Study [6] followed 12,000 men aged between 40 and 50 years for 10 years and reported a strong relationship between a serum cholesterol level of above 5.7 mmol/l and the development of CHD. Those with a cholesterol level above 7.75 mmol/l had a 3 times greater risk of myocardial infarction than those with a level of 5.8 mmol/l or less. Similar results were reported by the Pooling Research Group in the USA [7]. Although serum cholesterol and incidence of CHD are correlated between populations, there are differences in CHD rates that cannot be explained in this way. Thus, average serum cholesterol is only slightly higher in Scotland than in France while CHD mortality is 4 times more common among Scots men [8]. This does not appear to be due to underdiagnosis of CHD in France. There can also be considerable differences in CHD rates in communities. There is, for example, marked variation in coronary mortality between men in Glasgow and Edinburgh:

| | Cholesterol, mmol/l | Coronary SMR |
|---|---|---|
| Edinburgh | 6.4 | 81 |
| North Glasgow | 6.3 | 117 |

Measurement of the lipid-bearing fractions of plasma by ultracentrifugation has provided more detailed evidence of both the harmful and the possible protective role of these particles in CHD.

The main lipoprotein fractions are: (a) chylomicrons; (b) very low density lipoprotein (VLDL); (c) low density lipoprotein (LDL), and (d) high density lipoprotein (HDL).

The risk of CHD appears to rise most definitely with increased LDL levels. HDL, on the other hand, may have a protective effect [9]. Exercise and a moderate alcohol intake can both increase HDL levels. There has been controversy over the role of triglyceride, transported from the gut to the liver as chylomicrons and from the liver to peripheral tissues as VLDL. Triglyceride levels are positively correlated with total cholesterol, obesity, diabetes and have been difficult to assess as an independent risk factor. There has however been renewed interest in raised triglyceride levels especially in conjunction with low HDL levels [10]. There may well be an increased risk of CHD in this situation. Measurements of VLDL turnover following a fatty meal also show differences in the presence of established CHD [11].

There seems overall agreement that perturbations of lipid metabolism are implicated in the development of atherosclerosis and of vascular disease. Their importance must not be overemphasized and certainly many other factors are involved. Nonetheless, reduction of cholesterol levels, in both primary and secondary prevention studies, has been shown to decrease the incidence of CHD events, although there has been no change in total mortality. Vigorous treatment of raised cholesterol has also been shown angiographically to slow the progression of atherosclerosis and perhaps even to regress established lesions [12].

### *Plasma Fibrinogen*

A raised plasma fibrinogen is now recognized as an important risk factor for CHD [13]. It has also the theoretical attraction of providing a link between CHD, atherosclerosis and the coagulation system. Raised triglyceride levels are also associated with increased fibrinogen and those with a high cholesterol and high fibrinogen may be at particular risk [14]. Exercise increases fibrinolytic activity but no pharmacological modifications of fibrinogen reduction have as yet been assessed for their effect on CHD incidence.

### *Age, Sex and Heredity*

These are all important cardiovascular risk factors, immutable though they are. In all populations studied, men have higher rates than women, the incidence increases with age and those with a family history of premature vascular disease have themselves a greater risk of disease (which is not necessarily related to cholesterol levels). It has usually been assumed that CHD risk data and the results of intervention studies can be extrapolated to women. This may not be so. Isles et al. [15] have reported that women have lower CHD rates despite higher levels of cholesterol. It is also known that CHD rates do rise after the menopause but remain lower than men of a similar age. Oestrogen may still have a protective role beyond the time of menopause.

### *Hypertension*

Raised blood pressure is a major risk factor for CHD. The gradient of risk rises steeply and occurs in both men and women [4, 16]. Even minor differences appear to be important and confirm what insurance companies have practised for years in terms of 'loading' policies for life insurance. McMahon et al. [17] have reported that a difference as small as 6 mm Hg diastolic pressure was associated with 22% fewer fatal and non-fatal myocardial infarctions and 36% fewer strokes. A raised systolic pressure is also now known to carry the same ominous prognosis as does diastolic pressure.

The risks of raised blood pressure are well established. What is disappointing is that reduction of raised pressure has only very slightly reduced the risk. A meta-analysis [18] involving 37,000 individuals, 1,400 CHD events and 700 strokes found that the overall risk of CHD was reduced by 12% (confidence limits 0–20%) whereas there was a highly significant 43% reduction in the risk of stroke. There are several possible explanations. There has been speculation that too great a reduction in blood pressure might be associated with an increased mortality from CHD – perhaps due to reduced coronary perfusion pressure. Overall, however, mortality rates appear to be continuous rather than 'J' shaped. It has also been suggested that a new set of risks may be introduced by antihypertensive therapy, thus reducing the benefits of blood pressure control. Minor increases in triglyceride and cholesterol levels by diuretics and by non-selective $\beta$-blocking drugs might be relevant. It seems sensible to measure cholesterol as part of the initial assessment and adapt therapy by consideration of these results.

### *The Multiple Risk Factor Approach*

It is facile to expect that control of a single risk factor will be adequate to reduce the clinical burden of CHD. CHD is a multifactorial disease demanding a multifactorial approach. In the American Pooling Project [7] men aged between 30–59 years who smoked cigarettes doubled the risk of myocardial infarction. The combination of raised cholesterol ($>$6.5 mmol/l) and raised diastolic blood pressure ($>$90 mm Hg) increased the risk of infarction 4 times. Those who smoked had raised cholesterol and raised blood pressure increased their risk 8-fold. Some risk factors (age, sex, heredity) are obviously non-modifiable. All the more reason therefore for the individual to modify avoidable risks and for the physician to be in a position to offer appropriate advice. There is evidence that advice on diet, smoking, obesity, blood pressure and exercise can be beneficial and effective in some populations [19]. Such an approach should be widely adopted.

### *References*

1 Ross R, Glomsett JA: The pathogenesis of atherosclerosis. N Engl J Med 1976;25:369–377.

2 World Health Organisation: Prevention of coronary heart disease. Tech Rep Ser No 678. Geneva, WHO, 1982.

3 Nicholls ES, Jung J, Davies JW: Cardiovascular disease mortality in Canada. Can Med Assoc J 1981;125:981–992.

4 Shaper AG, Pocock SJ, Walker M, Phillips AM, Whitehead TP, Macfarlane PW: Risk factors for ischaemic heart disease: The prospective phase of the British Regional Heart Study. J Epidemiol Community Health 1985;39:197–209.

5 Castelli WP: Epidemiology of coronary heart disease: The Framingham Study. American Journal of Medicine Symposium, Feb 1984, pp 4–12.

6 Keys A: Coronary disease in seven countries. Circulation 1970;42(suppl 1):1–221.

7 Pooling Project Research Group: Relation of blood pressure, serum cholesterol, smoking habit, relative weight and ECG abnormalities to incidence of major coronary events. J Chronic Dis 1978;31:201–306.

8 Tunstall-Pedoe H, Smith WCS, Crombie IK: Levels and trends of coronary heart disease mortality in Scotland compared with other countries. Health Bull 1986;44:152–161.

9 Watkins LO, Neaton JD, Kuller LH (for the MRFIT Research Group): High density lipoprotein cholesterol and coronary heart disease incidence in black and white MRFIT usual care men. Circulation 1985;71:417A.

10 Castelli WP: The triglyceride issue: A view from Framingham. Am Heart J 1986;112(2):432–437.

11 Simpson HS, Williamson CM, Olivecrona T, Pringle S, McLean J, Lorimer AR, Bonnefous F, Bogaievsky Y, Packard CJ, Shepherd J: Post-prandial lipaemia: Fenofibrate and coronary heart disease. Atherosclerosis 1990;85:193–202.

12 Blankenhorn DH, Nessim SA, Johnson RL, Sanmarco ME, Azon SP, Casmin-Hemphill L: Beneficial effects of combined colestipol-niacin therapy on coronary atherosclerosis and coronary venous bypass grafts. JAMA 1987;257:3233–3240.

13 Meads TW, Mellows S, Brozovic M, Miller GJ, Chakrabarti RR, North WR, Haines AP, Sterling Y, Imeson JD, Thompson SG: Haemostatic function and ischaemic heart disease: Principal results of the Northwick Park Heart Study. Lancet 1986;ii:533–537.

14 Stone MC, Thorp JM: Plasma fibrinogen – A major coronary risk factor. JR Coll Gen Pract 1985;35:565–569.

15 Isles CG, Hole DJ, Gillis CR, Hawthorne VM, Lever AF: Plasma cholesterol, coronary heart disease and cancer in the Renfrew and Paisley Survey. BMJ 1989;298:920–924.

16 Kannell WB, Neaton JD, Wentworth D, Thomas HE, Stamler J, Hulley SB, Kjelsberg MO: Overall and coronary heart disease mortality rates in relation to major risk factors in 325,348 men screened for the MRFIT. Am Heart J 1986;112:825–836.

17 McMahon S, Peto R, Cutler J: Blood pressure, stroke and coronary heart disease. 1. Prolonged differences in blood pressure. Prospective observational studies corrected for regression dilution bias. Lancet 1990;335:765–774.

18 Collins R, Peto R, McMahon S, Herbert P, Fiebach NH, Eberlain KA, Godwin J, Qizilbash N, Taylor JO, Hennekens CH: Blood pressure, stroke and coronary heart disease. 2. Short-term reduction in blood pressure. Overview of randomised drug trials in their epidemiological context. Lancet 1990;335:827–838.

19 WHO European Collaborative Group: European collaborative trial of multifactorial prevention of coronary heart disease: Final report on the 6-year results. Lancet 1986;i:869–872.


A.R. Lorimer, Honorary Professor in Medicine, Royal Infirmary,
Glasgow G31 2ER (UK)

# Mechanisms

Weetman DF, Wood D (eds): Risk Factors for Cardiovascular Disease in Non-Smokers. Int. Workshop, Washington, Tyne and Wear, 1991. Basel, Karger, 1993, pp 7–15

## Cellular Events in the Development of Atherosclerosis

*Richard Bruckdorfer*

Department of Biochemistry and Chemistry, Royal Free Hospital School of Medicine, London, UK

Atherosclerosis (or atheroma) is an abnormal condition of blood vessels which underlies a number of clinical disorders of the vascular system including myocardial infarction, angina pectoris, arterial aneurysms, intermittent claudication and peripheral vascular disease. Genetic susceptibility may render certain individuals more vulnerable than others. There is a minority of cases where genetic predisposition clearly is the key cause, e.g. familial hypercholesterolaemia which in its heterzygous form will only affect about 1 in 500 of the population in the UK. The principal risk factors are considered to be elevated plasma cholesterol concentrations, hypertension and smoking which may, at least in part, be considered to be environmental in nature. In nonsmokers, hypercholesterolaemia and hypertension are the principal factors, although there are many other predisposing factors including obesity, diabetes, gender, exercise and diet to name just a few. Clearly there is an interaction of environmental and genetic factors.

### *The Development of Atherosclerosis*

The artery has a structure consisting (from the lumen outwards) of the endothelium, the elastic lamina, the media (smooth muscle) and adventitia. It is now clear that the endothelium is not an impermeable barrier and will allow even large molecules including lipoproteins to pass through, although the rates of movement are very different. There is considerable controversy over the precise sequence of the events leading to early atherosclerosis. A popular theory is that it arises as a result of injury to the artery wall and trauma to the endothelium, followed by movement or insudation of materials from the blood into the intima. It is uncertain what causes the initial damage to the endothelium and there may be a variety of agents. For example, mechanical damage in certain locations due to hypertension may be important since atherosclerosis is focal, particularly at branch points or where there is constant movement as is the case for coronary arteries. The damage may be chemical due to toxins or the high concentration of lipids or it may be immunological in origin. In cellular terms, the current emphasis is on an early appearance of blood monocytes which adhere to the endothelium and force themselves between the endothelial junctions into the intima, where they are activated and transformed into macrophages [1]. Early atherosclerotic plaques are characterized by the presence of significantly increased numbers of macrophages. The macrophages are capable of accumulating large amounts of lipid which leads to the formation of foam cells which carry most of the intracellular lipid (mainly cholesterol and cholesterol ester) in atherosclerotic plaque. Another important event is the stimulation of cellular proliferation at the early stage of atherosclerosis, particularly that of smooth muscle cells which may break through the elastic lamina and eventually form the main mass of the atherosclerotic plaque. These smooth muscle cells may dedifferentiate during proliferation and also become capable of lipid uptake.

Another event, which perhaps receives less attention, but may be of great importance, is the modification of the extracellular matrix. This matrix consists of a variety of substances, particularly the proteoglycans or glycosaminoglycans, the synthesis of which is increased following injury to the arterial wall. These substances, which are similar in structure to chondroitin sulphate, show increased sulphation after injury.

### *Plasma Lipoproteins*

Plasma lipoproteins, the normal function of which is to transport insoluble lipids from the gut or the liver to the periphery, or back to the liver [2], are thought to play an important role in the development of early atherosclerosis. It is therefore appropriate to look briefly at their properties at this stage.

The principal classes of lipoproteins, in increasing order of density, are chylomicrons, very-low-density lipoproteins (VLDL), low-density lipoproteins (LDL) and high-density lipoproteins (HDL). The density profile arises from the lipid content which is always greater as the density decreases and makes the classes readily separable by ultracentrifugation. It is important to recognize that each fraction is heterogeneous, containing a range of particles within a particular density range, but on the whole have a fairly consistent metabolic function and composition with respect to type of proteins they contain.

The least dense classes (chylomicrons and VLDL) have a large percentage of triacylglycerol and less cholesterol, whereas those of higher density (LDL and HDL) have little triacylglycerol but are rich in cholesterol. LDL are the principal carriers of cholesterol.

Apolipoprotein B (apoB) is the sole protein of the LDL fraction and is so large that there is only one molecule per LDL particle which contains 3,000–4,000 lipid molecules. This gave rise to the discovery by Brown and Goldstein [3] of high-affinity receptors for apoB on the plasma membrane, initially on fibroblasts, but later on most cell types. The primary function of this receptor is the uptake of LDL into the cell and consequently the removal of cholesterol from the circulation. The effect of this is two-fold. Firstly, cholesterol biosynthesized in the liver is delivered to extrahepatic cells and may be used in resynthesis of membranes, especially during cell division. Secondly, it is a mechanism by which cholesterol from the periphery is returned to the liver, since about 60–70% of the receptor activity is located in the liver. The key role for these receptors is very evident in patients with familial hypercholesterolaemia, a genetic disorder where the receptor is absent or defective. The high concentrations of LDL in the circulation predispose the patients to premature myocardial infarction. Other receptors have been described which can also bind and internalize LDL and related particles. In macrophages, there are receptors called scavenger receptors which will avidly bind and take up LDL which have been modified by reactions with the positively charged amino acids lysine and arginine. Such modifications take place during the oxidation of LDL (see below). The macrophage has very little capacity to bind the native LDL, but the scavenger receptors bind and internalize the oxidatively modified LDL [4].

### *The Oxidative Modification of LDL and Atherosclerosis*

Incubation of LDL with isolated or cultured cells, such as endothelial cells, macrophages or smooth muscle cells, enhances the oxidation of the lipoproteins so that they are no longer recognized by the high-affinity receptors, but are taken up by the macrophage scavenger receptors. The oxidation involves the degradation of polyunsaturated fatty acids, the formation of lysolecithin and the modification of the apoB as measured by disappearance of available lysine. These changes can be mimicked by simple incubations with transition metal ions such as cupric or ferrous ions. The cells are known to release reactive oxygen species and free radicals as part of their normal metabolism and it is suggested that if the passage of LDL through the artery wall is retarded, perhaps due to the presence of high concentrations of LDL below the endothelium or due to sequestration by sulphate or other groups on the glycosaminoglycans of the extracellular matrix, the oxidative process proceeds and may unleash the pathophysiological processes leading to the formation of foam cells characteristic of atherosclerosis [5]. LDL normally carry a number of lipid-soluble antioxidants of dietary origin such as a vitamin E or plant carotenoids. It is possible that the LDL may be protected from oxidation by the presence of these and water-soluble antioxidants such as ascorbate. Studies in vitro show that these antioxidants are the first to disappear after an oxidative challenge before the breakdown of the fatty acids commences. It is interesting that in a study in Edinburgh [6] both low plasma vitamin E and C concentrations were related to the occurrence of chest pain due to angina pectoris. Similar relationships have been found in cross-sectional studies of a number of European countries with widely differing incidences of cardiovascular disease.

The mechanism of oxidation in vivo is still not clear and, as indicated above, the origin of the oxidation not identified. One proposal is that the LDL needs to be 'seeded' with peroxides which are always found in small amounts in isolated lipoproteins. Over a number of decades there have been reports of the accumulation of lipid peroxides in atherosclerotic tissue and of lysolecithin in high concentrations. In the last few years, considerable efforts have been made to try and locate modified lipoproteins in the arterial wall and this has been achieved with the use of fluorescently labelled antibodies to oxidized LDL [7]. Naturally-occurring antibodies are also found in the circulation of some individuals, especially those with cardiovascular disease. It is supposed that these may have arisen in response to the release of oxidized LDL, or its more mature form known to the pathologists as ceroid, from fissures in advanced atherosclerotic plaques [8]. Furthermore, LDL obtained from rabbit atherosclerotic plaques not only show a strong similarity to LDL oxidized in vitro, but also react with polyclonal antibodies which recognize oxidized LDL.

It has long been recognized that cytotoxic products resulting from the oxidation of lipids will destroy cells or impair their function. These effects are now considered to have potential importance in the development of atherosclerosis. It is probable that differing cell types are affected by different products of lipoprotein oxidation. Some of these products also have potent chemotactic properties. Oxidized LDL increases monocyte adhesion to the endothelium, one of the earliest events in the development of atherosclerosis [9]. In addition to attracting monocytes to the site of the damage (and where modification of the lipoproteins has occurred) oxidized

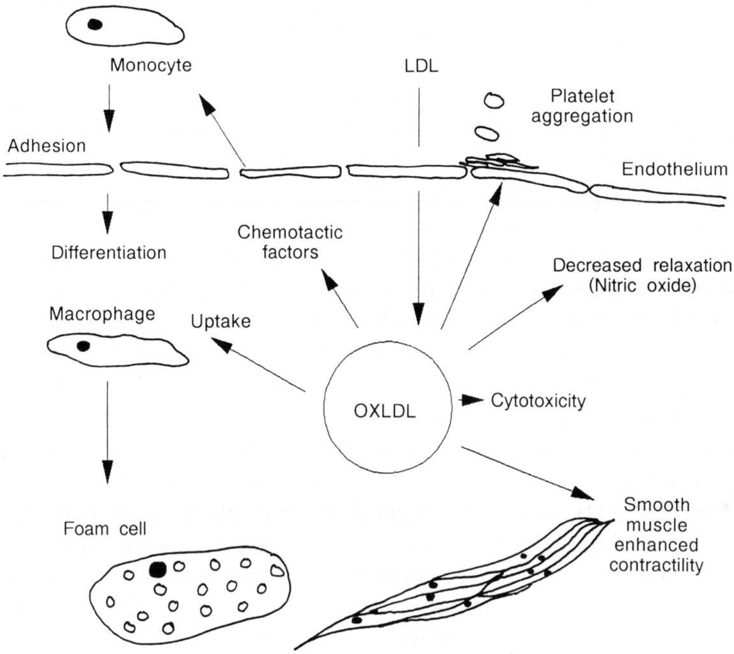


*Fig. 1.* The influence of oxidation of LDL on cellular processes in atherosclerosis and thrombosis.

LDL also inhibits the departure of macrophages from the site of the lesion, therefore interfering with the role of the macrophage in removing unwanted materials from the damaged area. Figure 1 summarizes the influence of oxidized LDL on the cellular processes described above and below.

### *Later Stages in Atherosclerosis*

As indicated above, the early stages in atherosclerosis, although important to our understanding of the disease, may not have a great deal of significance in clinical events. The maturing of the plaque results from repeated insults to the endothelium and subendothelial tissue, takes many years and often occurs only in specific locations, for example in one or more branches of the coronary arteries or in the femoral artery. The increased plaque size introduces new factors which are potentially life-threatening. The thickening of the artery wall leads to problems of nutrient and oxygen supply which results in tissue necrosis. The weakened wall may 'bubble' outwards or the necrotic material burst into the lumen of the artery with catastrophic results. Such events are highly likely to result in thrombosis which accompanies a very high proportion of myocardial events. The resulting ischaemia and subsequent events bring about the damage to the myocardium, the extent of which determines the likelihood of death. In angina pectoris, severe atherosclerosis is also an important contributory factor in most cases and sometimes foreshadows later infarction. However, in this case there is no obvious platelet involvement and it may involve the contraction of the atherosclerotic arteries under conditions of exercise or stress or following other unrecognized stimuli. Therefore the clinical events frequently depend on reductions in blood flow because of changes in vascular tone or because of thrombosis.

Platelets are activated by their exposure to collagen, which may become exposed if there is a break in the endothelium, or by the release of other substances such as ADP. The first indications that platelets may be sensitized by LDL was the observation that platelets in patients with familial hypercholesterolaemia are more sensitive to platelet agonists. This was later confirmed by a large study of 150 apparently healthy individuals where there was a strong relationship between plasma LDL concentration and platelet sensitivity to adrenaline and ADP. However, LDL which had been oxidized were more effective than native LDL in sensitizing platelets [10]. Since fissures in complex atherosclerotic plaques are known to occur and are likely to be the site of thrombus formation, oxidized LDL may contribute to the activation of the platelet at this point.

The endothelium provides a surface which is antithrombotic and produces substances which also regulate vascular tone. Both surfaces of the endothelium are exposed to high concentrations of lipoproteins, especially LDL. In atherosclerosis, LDL in the intima may be oxidized, either partially or severely, and cause cytotoxic damage to the endothelium. The vascular endothelium releases a factor, previously called endothelium-derived relaxing factor (EDRF) which inhibits platelet aggregation and causes relaxation of smooth muscle if it has been previously contracted by agents such as noradrenaline or serotonin. These effects are mediated by the release of nitric oxide or a labile nitroso-compound from the endothelium. A sensitive indicator of endothelial damage appears to be a dysfunction in relaxation mediated by EDRF. There is increasing evidence that in human coronary arteries, impairment of the vasomotor responses to endothelium-dependent vasodilators may precede angiographic evidence of atherosclerotic lesions [11]. A recent study has shown that in hypercholesterolaemic patients with elevated plasma LDL, endothelium-dependent relaxation is progressively impaired as atherosclerosis develops [12]. Exposure of rings of arterial tissue to LDL in the organ bath mimicks the impairment found in hypercholesterolaemia. Native LDL exerts an inhibition on endothelium-dependent relaxation. Inhibition by oxidatively modified LDL is more intense [13].

As mentioned earlier, smooth muscle cells also are capable of oxidizing LDL and developing into foam cells. In addition, atherosclerosis enhances the contraction of smooth muscle. There is now evidence that oxidized lipoproteins enhance the contraction of endothelium-denuded arteries by serotonin which will increase the tendency to vasoconstriction [14].

In conclusion, there are many aspects of the lifelong process of development of atherosclerosis which are not yet understood or their relative importance fully appreciated. Certain theories achieve prominence and then wane, possibly to be resurrected later as new evidence is brought forward.

## *References*


1 Ross R: The pathogenesis of atherosclerosis – an update. N Engl J Med 1986;314:488–500.

2 Durrington PN: Hyperlipidaemia: Diagnosis and Management. London, Butterworths, 1989, pp 23–55.

3 Brown MS, Goldstein ML: A receptor-mediated pathway for cholesterol homeostasis. Science 1986;232:34–47.

4 Mahley RW, Innerarity TI, Weisgraber KH, Oh SO: Altered metabolism (in vivo and in vitro) of plasma lipoproteins after selective chemical modification of lysine residues of the apoproteins. J Clin Invest 1979;64:743–750.

5 Steinberg D, Witztum JL: Lipoproteins and atherogenesis – current concepts. J Am Med Assoc 1990;264:3047–3052.

6 Riemersma RA, Wood DA, Macintyre CC, Elton R, Gey KF, Oliver MF: Low plasma vitamins E and C. Increased risk of angina in Scottish men. Ann NY Acad Sci 1989;570:291–295.

7 Yla Herttuala S, Palinski W, Rosenfeld ME, Parthasarathy S, Carew TE, Butler S, Witztum JL, Steinberg D: Evidence for the presence of oxidatively modified low density lipoprotein in atherosclerotic lesions of rabbit and man. J Clin Invest 1989;84:1086–1095.

8 Mitchinson MJ, Ball RY, Carpenter KLH, Parums DV: Macrophages and ceroid in atherosclerosis; in Suckling KE, Groot PE (eds): Hyperlipidaemias and Atherosclerosis. London, Academic Press, 1988, pp 117–134.

9 Cushing SD, Berliner JA, Valente AJ, Territo MC, Navab M, Parhami F, Gerrity R, Schwartz CJ, Fogelman AM: Minimally modified low density lipoprotein induces monocyte chemotactic protein 1 in human endothelial and smooth muscle cells. Proc Natl Acad Sci USA 1990;87:5134–5138.

10 Bruckdorfer KR: The effects of plasma lipoproteins on platelet responsiveness and on platelet and vascular prostanoid synthesis. Prostaglandins Leukot Essent Fatty Acids 1989;38:247–254.

11 Vita JA, Treasure CB, Nabel EG, McLenachen JM, Fish RD, Yeung AC, Vekshtein

VD, Selwyn AP, Ganz P: Coronary vasomotor response to acetylcholine relates to risk factors for coronary artery disease. Circulation 1990;81:491–497.
12 Zeiher AM, Drexler H, Wollschlager H, Just H: Modulation of coronary vasomotor tone in humans – progressive endothelial dysfunction with different early stages of coronary atherosclerosis. Circulation 1991;83:391–401.
13 Jacobs M, Plane F, Bruckdorfer KR: Native and oxidised low-density lipoproteins have different inhibitory effects on endothelium-derived relaxing factor in the rabbit aorta. Br J Pharmacol 1990;100:21–26.
14 Galle J, Bassenge E, Busse R: Oxidised low density lipoproteins potentiate vasoconstrictions to various agonists by direct interaction with vascular smooth muscle. Circ Res 1990;66:1287–1293.

Dr. Richard Bruckdorfer, Department of Biochemistry and Chemistry,
Royal Free Hospital School of Medicine, London NW3 2PF (UK)

## *Discussion*

*Butlin* (Sunderland): The finding of atherosclerotic lesions in the blood vessels of the young is interesting. Is there evidence that the incidence of this is increasing?

*Bruckdorfer* (London): The pathologists know more about this, but these lesions seem to appear and disappear, and can only be observed if children die for other reasons. I do not know of any statistics indicating that they are becoming more common: perhaps they are becoming less likely now that neonatal and childhood nutrition is better understood. The 'war babies' are now of an age where they are at risk of atherosclerosis and perhaps the slight decline in incidence is due to the restricted diet in their early, formative years, although I know of no direct evidence for this.

*X:* In your model, you showed LDL becoming oxidized after crossing the endothelial cell. Is there evidence for oxidized LDL in plasma or that LDL can be oxidized by endothelial cells themselves?

*Bruckdorfer:* There is great debate about whether oxidized LDL is found in plasma. Lipid peroxides are found in plasma and are elevated in certain groups such as diabetics. VLDL is increased in diabetics and this is also susceptible to oxidation, but probably less gets through the endothelium. There is evidence for oxidized lipoproteins inside the artery wall: fluorescently labelled antibodies to oxidized lipoprotein and to LDL itself indicate that these compounds are only found in the artery wall in the region of atherosclerosis. Dr. Mitchinson at Cambridge has found circulating naturally-occurring antibodies to ceroid which cross-react with oxidized LDL (ceroid can be regarded as a mature form of oxidized LDL). In Italy, Avogaro et al. [Arteriosclerosis 1988;8:79–87] have also reported oxidized LDL in the circulation. If oxidized too far, reticuloendothelial cells of the liver will recognize and remove it. If it is there in plasma, then it must only be marginally oxidized LDL. There is evidence that marginally oxidized LDL, where only a little of the lipid is changed and the protein is not affected, could be highly cytotoxic and chemotactic.

*Roe* (Wimbledon): Is there evidence that introduction and proper use of insulin pumps has cut down incidence of peripheral vascular disease in diabetics? If so, might this imply that the insulin deficiency rather than glucose excess is the risk factor?

*Bruckdorfer:* The theory is that good control of diabetes decreases the secondary risks, but I do not know any evidence about pumps. In the nondiabetic population, individuals with slight glucose intolerance show an increased risk of cardiovascular diseases, indicating that poor glucose control may lead to increased risk. I did not mention that LDL and probably VLDL can be nonenzymatically glycosylated at high glucose concentrations. There is some suggestion that glycosylated LDL can be handled rather like oxidized LDL and may be more likely to stick on to the extracellular matrix of the arterial wall, so this is a biochemical reason why glucose may be a risk factor.

*Roe:* Perhaps people interested in diabetes concentrated too much on glucose level, which might be relatively harmless, and too little on circulating insulin which is definitely required for proper metabolism?

*Bruckdorfer:* There is a suggestion that insulin exacerbates lipid metabolism in the arterial wall, but there is insufficient evidence to be certain. To be Asian in the UK is a risk factor: Bengalis in east London have 50% higher risk than the indigenous population of cardiovascular disease, and the risk relates to the higher prevalence of diabetes amongst the Asian group.

*X:* A high proportion of the fatty acids in LDL is polyunsaturated, the vast majority coming via LCAT (lecithin cholesterol acyl transferase). Is there evidence for variation in the proportion of unsaturates and if so does this relate to the susceptibility of LDL to oxidation?

*Bruckdorfer:* Dr. Steinberg, who is the author of these oxidation theories, has fed rabbits on sunflower oil in which the usual linoleic acid has been replaced by oleic acid. Compared with rabbits fed normal sunflower oil, their LDL was less susceptible to oxidation. Similar studies are being carried out in humans. This result fits in with the current idea that monounsaturates are at least as or more cardioprotective than polyunsaturates. If the diet contains unsaturates, it nearly always contains antioxidants from fresh fruit and vegetables as well, whereas with a diet containing much hard fat this may not be so.

Weetman DF, Wood D (eds): Risk Factors for Cardiovascular Disease in Non-Smokers. Int. Workshop, Washington, Tyne and Wear, 1991. Basel, Karger, 1993, pp 16–23

# Physiological Regulation of the Cardiovascular System: Implications for Sudden Death and Other Cardiovascular Conditions

*A.G. Ramage*

Department of Pharmacology, Royal Free Hospital Medical School, London, UK

The condition of sudden death results from sudden ventricular fibrillation and is responsible for approximately 70,000 deaths per year in the UK. An interesting feature of this condition is that patients who have been resuscitated following an episode of sudden fibrillation may continue to live for a prolonged period without further episodes. Additionally, the occurrence of sudden death is not correlated with other cardiovascular pathologies, such as degree of atheroma [1], and thus the underlying cause is undefined. Two groups of factors may give rise to ventricular fibrillation, loss of cardiac output and death: these are neuronal factors and ischaemic factors. Ishaemic factors are considered elsewhere, and this contribution will concentrate on neuronal factors involved in the physiological control of the cardiovascular system and will consider those aspects of behavioural activity which could potentially lead to ventricular fibrillation via a physiological rather than a pathophysiological mechanism.

The activity of the heart is influenced by both the sympathetic and the parasympathetic divisions of the autonomic nervous system. Sympathetic stimulation increases the force and rate of the heart and increases oxygen consumption by the myocardium. Parasympathetic stimulation slows the heart, so reducing oxygen demand, and can stop the heart. Excessive sympathetic or excessive parasympathetic stimulation can occur in response to everyday activities and may result in ventricular fibrillation: each will be considered separately.

## *Excessive Sympathetic Stimulation of the Heart*

The sympathetic nerves supplying the heart mediate effects predominantly by releasing noradrenaline which activates $\beta$-adrenoceptors. $\beta$-adrenoceptor antagonists have been shown to reduce the incidence of

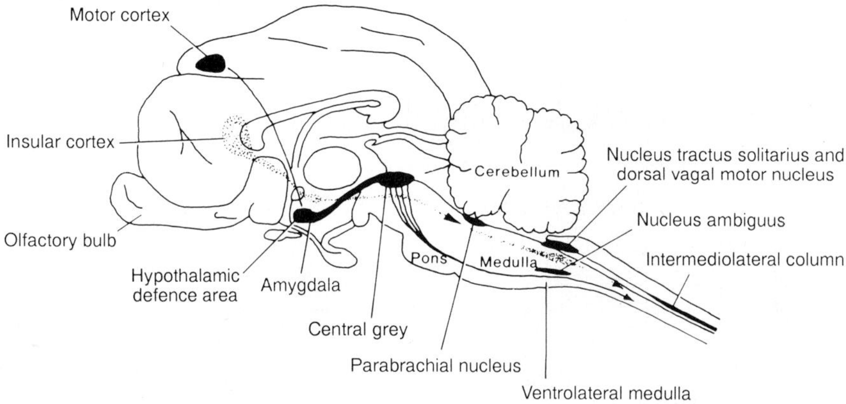


*Fig. 1.* Paramedial sagittal section through the brain to show areas which are important in central control of cardiovascular function.

sudden death in high risk patients who have survived acute myocardial infarction [2], perhaps suggesting that overactivity of the sympathetic nerve supply in certain situations may cause the condition by provoking cardiac arrhythmias.

Increased sympathetic drive occurs normally as part of the defence reaction, an alerting reaction to threatening stimuli such as being interviewed, lecturing and being threatened by sabre-tooth tigers. This reaction involves tachycardia, hypertension, vasoconstriction in blood vessels supplying the skin, gastrointestinal tract and kidneys and vasodilation in blood vessels of skeletal muscles, providing good blood flow to active muscle groups. Another important component of this reaction is that the baroreceptor reflex arc, which normally ensures tight control of blood pressure, is overridden by the central nervous system so that the blood pressure can rise dramatically and thus maintain good perfusion of skeletal muscle beds.

The behavioural and cardiovascular components of the defence reaction can be provoked by stimulating the hypothalamic defence area in the brain (fig. 1) [3]. The nearby amygdala, which is part of the limbic system, provides an afferent input to the hypothalamus and plays an important role in the integration of the cardiovascular changes associated with emotion, including an alerting reaction. More generally, pathways involved in the integration of cardiovascular responses include the ventromedial area of the medulla (concerned with vasomotor control), the nucleus tractus solitarius, which is the terminal area for the afferent nerves from the baroreceptors, and the dorsal vagal motor nucleus, which is the origin of vagal fibres innervating the heart.

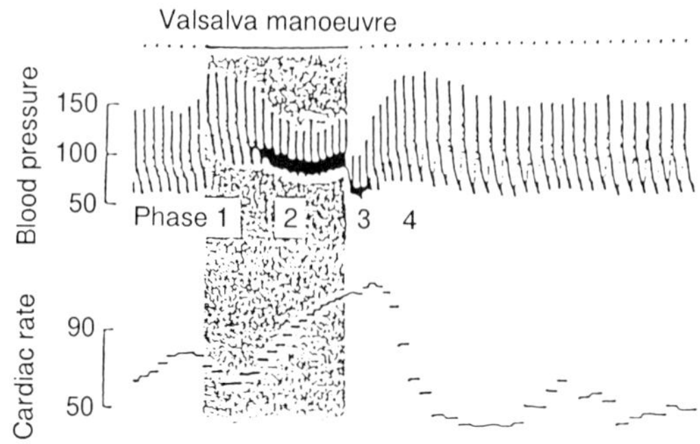


*Fig. 2.* Cardiovascular changes occurring during and after the Valsalva manoeuvre (forced expiration against a closed or narrow glottis). Adapted from [7].

Whereas in man the defence reaction is an alerting, sympathetic response, it is interesting that in other species such as rabbit the defence reaction may involve 'playing dead' or freezing when threatened. This is considered a vagal, parasympathetic response, involving hypotension and bradycardia, which may be severe [4].

Another important and common physiological activity which affects the cardiovascular system is the Valsalva manoeuvre. This is a maintained and forced expiration against a closed or narrow glottis, such as may be employed when straining to defecate. The cardiovascular response to this manoeuvre provides a useful test of autonomic function in man. Forced expiration increases intrathoracic pressure and compresses the vena cava, so that initially blood is pushed into the heart, the cardiac output rises and therefore the blood pressure rises (phase 1, fig. 2). But venous return to the heart has been decreased and soon cardiac output and blood pressure fall (phase 2). This provokes a pronounced tachycardia brought about by baroreceptor reflex. In phase 3, immediately after release of the forced expiration, the blood pressure falls and heart rate rises slightly, but then blood pressure rises markedly due to increased venous return and this provokes a reflex fall in heart rate during phase 4.

In addition to defecating, coughing, lifting heavy weights, playing a high resistance instrument such as the trumpet, singing high notes, or indulging in coitus can all induce the same pattern of changes. The marked tachycardia during phase 2 could provide excessive sympathetic stimulation of the heart and might precipitate arrhythmias and lead to sudden death.

*Excessive Parasympathetic Stimulation of the Heart*

The parasympathetic supply to the heart is provided by the vagus (tenth cranial) nerves. There are a number of situations in which the vagus nerves become active and the most obvious effect is to slow down the rate of the heart.

The influence of the vagus nerves on the heart can be seen by studying heart rate during normal respiration. Cardiac vagal motoneurones are found in the nucleus ambiguus (fig. 1) and provide background vagal tone to the heart, slowing it. Neurones controlling respiration are located around the area of the nucleus ambiguus. At each inspiration, heart rate increases because the background activity in the vagal motor nerves is inhibited by the activity in the inspiratory neurones. This fluctuation in heart rate with respiration is called sinus arrhythmia: the rate may fluctuate by 5% during normal quiet breathing and by as much as 30% during laboured respiration. If respiration is inhibited, this interaction is lost and there is no protection against excessive activation of cardiac vagal motoneurones. Hence, excessive slowing of the heart may occur.

Before considering situations in which respiration is inhibited (either deliberately or accidentally) it is necessary to review the role of peripheral chemoreceptors in respiratory and cardiovascular control. These are located in the aortic and carotid bodies (fig. 3) and they detect changes in the levels of oxygen, carbon dioxide and hydrogen ions in the blood bathing the bodies. A fall in oxygen level and rises in carbon dioxide and hydrogen ion levels. e.g. in hypoxia or in haemorrhagic hypotension, result in stimulation of respiration. Under such conditions, impulses are also sent to the vasomotor centre, which is excited, and there is a reflex elevation of arterial pressure by vasoconstriction (to maintain perfusion) and a bradycardia (to reduce oxygen consumption) in addition to stimulation of respiration (to promote exchange of gases). Thus the essential organs are protected.

Moving on to consider situations in which respiration is inhibited and the peripheral chemoreceptors may also come into play, the diving response is an excellent example [5]. This is a rapid response to immersion of the head and it is seen in all mammals. The response involves apnoea, pronounced vagally-induced bradycardia and sympathetic vasoconstriction, so that arterial pressure is maintained. It is prolonged in diving mammals, which can remain immersed for 1–2 h. The response can also be elicited by stimulation of sensory receptors on the face, at the back of the mouth, in the nose and in the pharynx, the afferent impulses travelling in the trigeminal and glossopharyngeal nerves to the medulla.

If apnoea is prolonged, it may give rise to hypoxia in the blood bathing the carotid and aortic bodies, which will induce a chemoreceptor

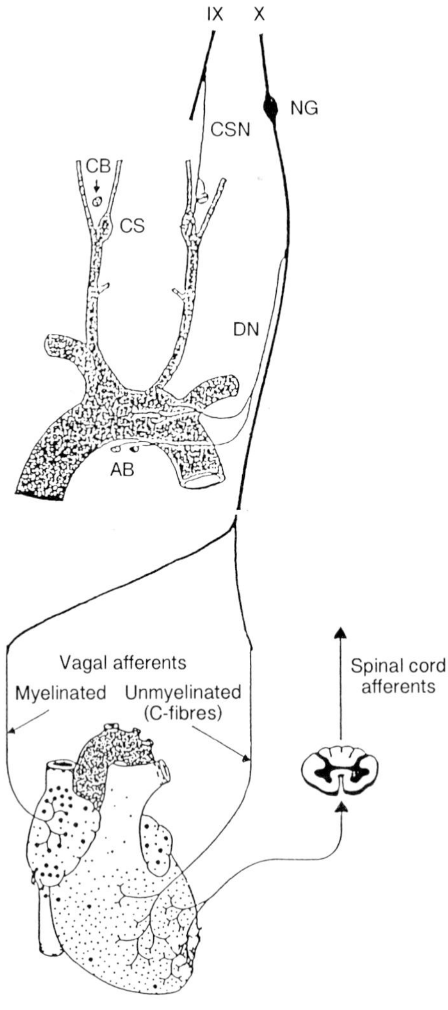


*Fig. 3.* Location of peripheral chemoreceptors and baroreceptors. CB = Carotid body; CS = carotid sinus; CSN = carotid sinus nerve; NG = nodose ganglia; AB = aortic bodies; DN = aortic nerve.

reflex. This may restart breathing, but if not, bradycardia induced through the carotid body chemoreceptor reflex could summate with the pronounced bradycardia of the diving response: this in the absence of the normal respiratory inhibition of cardiac vagal motoneurones. Excessive slowing of the heart could then result in cardiac arrest in certain situations.

*Table 1.* Cardiorespiratory interactions involving carotid bodies and upper airways receptors (after Daly and Angell-James [5])

| | |
|---|---|
| Clinical implications | |
| Bradycardia and cardiac arrest | |
| Surgical interventions | Nose |
| | Irrigation of sinuses |
| | Intubation, extubation |
| Laryngoscopy, bronchoscopy | |
| Asphyxia in quadriplegics | |
| Blackout in underwater swimmers | |
| Sleep apnoea syndromes | |
| A. Central | Bulbar poliomyelitis |
| | Ondine's curse |
| | Shy-Drager syndrome |
| | Drug intoxication |
| | Sudden infant death syndrome (cot death) |
| | Pierre-Robin syndrome |
| | Pickwickian syndrome |
| B. Obstructive | Pickwickian syndrome |
| | Adenoidal hypertrophy-pulm., hypertension syndrome |
| | Apnoea-stridor-bradycardia |
| | Syndrome of spina bifida |
| | Bird-like face syndrome |
| | (Dystrophia myotonica) |
| Restaurant or 'steak' deaths | |
| 'Sniffing' deaths | |
| Asthma deaths and pressurized aerosols | |

There are a number of situations in which these cardiorespiratory interactions may occur, mediated by chemoreceptors of the carotid and aortic bodies and the sensory receptors of the upper airways. These are circumstances in which bradycardia and cardiac arrest may ensue, giving them potential clinical importance [5]. Some are listed in table 1, including sudden infant death syndrome: these reflexes are particularly strong in neonates and the young compared with adult mammals.

Returning to figure 3, there is another reflex which involves the free nerve endings in the walls of the ventricle and the unmyelinated C-fibre afferents of the vagus. This is known as the cardiopulmonary reflex or the Von Bezold-Jarisch reflex. The sensory nerves are activated by ischaemia of the myocardium following occlusion of the coronary arteries, by changes in left ventricular end diastolic pressure and by changes in the inotropic state of the heart. The reflex response involves bradycardia, vasodilation and hypotension and is protective, preventing overwork of the heart. This reflex can be seen following inferoposterior myocardial ischaemia and infarction, during coronary arteriography, exertional syncope in aortic stenosis, vago-vagal syncope and heart failure [6]. A severe bradycardia may ensue, which can be avoided by treatment with atropine.

In summary, there is a series of cardiovascular conditions in which death is sudden and is due to the cessation of pumping activity by the heart but no common underlying pathology has been identified. Perhaps some clue can be found by considering the behavioural activities which influence the cardiovascular system and the physiological factors which normally control cardiovascular activity.

## *References*

1 Lown B: Sudden death from coronary heart disease; in Waldensatromy J, Larssons S, Ljungstedt C (eds): Skandid International Symposia. Early Phases of Coronary Heart Disease. Stockholm, Nordiska Bokhandelns Forlag, 1983, pp 255–277.
2 Beta-Blocker Heart Attack Study Group. J Am Med Assoc 1981;246:2073–2074.
3 Jordan D: Autonomic changes in affective behavior; in Loewy AD, Spyer KM (eds): Central regulation of autonomic functions. New York, Oxford University Press, 1990, pp 349–366.
4 Kapp BS, Pascoe JP, Bixler MA: The amygdala: a neuroanatomical systems approach to its contribution to aversive conditioning; in Buuters N, Squire LR (eds): The Neurophysiology of Memory. New York, Guilford Press, 1983, pp 473–488.
5 Daly M de B, Angell-James JE: The diving response, its clinical implications. Int Med 1979;1:12–19.
6 Mark AL: The Bezold-Jarisch reflex revisited: clinical implications of inhibitory reflexes originating in the heart. J Am Coll Cardiol 1983;1:90–102.
7 Bannister R: in Sleight P (ed): Arterial Blood Pressure and Hypertension. Oxford, Oxford University Press, 1980, pp 117–121.

Dr. A.G. Ramage, Department of Pharmacology, Royal Free Hospital Medical School, London NW3 2PF (UK)

## *Discussion*

*Weetman* (Sunderland): It is quite easy to demonstrate experimentally that when the vagus is stimulated, the heart stops. Then after a short wait the ventricles begin to beat without any contribution from the atrium – the classic vagal escape. How does that fit with the sort of cardiac arrest you have been describing?

*Ramage* (London): It could fit. We know that vagal escape does occur in excessive vagal stimulation, but perhaps if the stimulus is delivered at the wrong part of the beat, the heart may stop completely. Can vagal escape always be demonstrated experimentally?

*Weetman:* In my experience, yes.

*Ramage:* Yet situations obviously do occur where diving into water induces bradycardia with severe consequences.

*Werko* (Göteborg): It's possible that the subjects of your experiments were healthy, Prof. Weetman, whereas these individuals may have some sort of heart disease.

*Ramage:* Yes, when there is indication of underlying atheroma, but some people suffer sudden death when there is no obvious lesion. There may be a sudden arterial spasm, perhaps.

*Lee* (Sutton): Epidemiologists, when studying cardiovascular disease, normally measure generalized risk factors relating to the lifestyle of the patients. Do you think that they should routinely measure what the person was actually doing when he died of heart disease?

*Ramage:* Yes, I think they should, it could be interesting. I have tried to emphasize the behavioural problems and risk factors in this. The heart is strongly governed by the brain, and this is a factor which is often ignored.

*Armitage* (Knaresborough): You mentioned ventricular fibrillation at the beginning of your presentation and then discussed factors leading to cardiac arrest: after the heart has stopped, does it move into a fibrillation stage?

*Ramage:* I believe it does, although this is a question for the cardiologists, whereas my concern is with the physiological reflexes. Presumably there would be anoxia, the heart stopping for a certain period, other reflexes coming into play, giving excessive sympathetic stimulation with no blood flow and leading to fibrillation.

*Levy* (Birmingham): I was interested in what you said about sniffers and sudden death. In industry we've seen quite a few apparently healthy young men who have suddenly collapsed from cardiac arrest, who have been working with or near degreasing tanks of chlorinated hydrocarbons. Would these fit into your pattern?

*Ramage:* That would fit the vagal-diving response interaction, initiated by stimulation of the trigeminal nerve in these people. But how would you prove it and what drug would you give to prevent that reflex being switched in? It's an interesting problem.

*Levy:* The thought was that these people might have a pre-existing condition since many people are exposed to these substances but only some are affected. I think that nothing has been found in the pathology.

*Ramage:* We do know that hypertensives, for instance, seem to have a greater defence response for alerting stimulation compared with normal people. They may be genetically more prone to overreact to stressful situations.

Weetman DF, Wood D (eds): Risk Factors for Cardiovascular Disease in Non-Smokers. Int. Workshop, Washington, Tyne and Wear, 1991. Basel, Karger, 1993, pp 24–32

# Intracellular Mechanisms of Myocardial Infarction

*A. Markham* [1]

School of Health Sciences, University of Sunderland, Sunderland, UK

In the majority of patients with acute myocardial infarction coronary atherosclerosis is the underlying lesion preceding the infarct. The biochemical sequences leading to atherosclerotic plaques occur at different times in different individuals and that the plaques are of multifactorial origin [1], and set up biochemical consequences that are characteristic of myocardial ischaemia. The changes result from the myocardial oxygen demand exceeding that possible from the arterial blood, hence myocardial ischaemia develops. Under these circumstances the aerobic function of mitochondria, the organelles responsible for oxidative metabolism and adenosine triphosphate (ATP) biosynthesis, is markedly disrupted, so the formation of ATP falls dramatically [2–4].

Anaerobic glycolysis maintains a limited supply of ATP until the onset of end-product inhibition of the pathway. In this period the backup energy system of creatine phosphate is also reduced to approximately 20% of its normal level within 2 min of the infarction. In addition to the loss of high-energy phosphates, other cellular events contribute to a loss of myocardial cellular function during ischaemia; these include: (a) acidosis; (b) reduced sensitivity of contractile proteins to calcium ($Ca^{2+}$); (c) accumulation of phosphate and lipid; (d) enzyme release; (e) change in $Ca^{2+}$ homeostasis, and (f) radical formation and lipid peroxidation [5–8]. The overall effect of these intracellular changes is the rapid decline of systolic and diastolic function and the possibility of cell necrosis [9]. Thus the development of myocardial ischaemia can result in the cessation of normal systolic function within seconds [5].

Following cessation of coronary arterial blood flow, myocardial ischaemia appears first in the subendocardium, followed by a transmural

[1] The author wishes to thank Miss S.J. Jones for helping in the preparation of this document.

advance towards the subepicardium. The damage to ischaemic myocytes is believed to be reversible during this 15–20 min period; but from then onwards, the changes are of an irreversible nature, spreading through both the subendo- and subepicardium. Irreversible changes may be prevented if ATP levels remain $>70\%$ of control levels [10]. If myocardial blood flow is re-established, myocytes gradually replete adenine nucleotides; however, the return of normal systolic/diastolic function is inversely proportional to the duration of the ischaemic episode [11, 12]. The term 'stunned myocardium' has been used to describe such a severely, but reversibly, injured myocardium [13, 14].

Ischaemic episodes are almost always accompanied by some form of arrhythmia, which is detectable in the acute phase of myocardial infarction. Ventricular arrhythmias arise in the ischaemic peri-infarct zones and result from the following: (a) increased myocardial cell electrical automaticity; (b) slowing of conduction in specific areas of the heart with resultant re-entry and re-excitation loops, and (c) variable shortening or lengthening of the refactory period combined with increased dispersion of refractoriness between ischaemic and nonischaemic zones. In contrast, atrial arrhythmias are the result of the following: (a) ischaemic and/or necrosis of the arterial myocardium that is secondary to coronary thrombosis and (b) atrial dilatation due indirectly to elevated ventricular filling pressures. It should be noted that a wide array of atrial and/or ventricular arrhythmias can occur. These arrhythmias may be induced by known arrhythmogenic compounds that are released from the ischaemic myocardium, including cyclic AMP, free fatty acids, long chain fatty acids, lysophosphoglycerides, lactate and pyruvate. All the above compounds have electrophysiological activity [15].

Alterations in the metabolic processes associated with myocardial dysfunction are now known, in part, to relate to the dramatic changes in oxygen and $Ca^{2+}$ levels resulting from re-perfusion, usually referred to as the oxygen or $Ca^{2+}$ paradox [16]. In addition to oxygen or $Ca^{2+}$-induced toxicity, it should be noted that radiation, or the intracellular formation of one or more of the following unstable chemical species, may also initiate the onset of myocardial damage or dysfunction [9]: (a) electrophiles, which are commonly formed from C-, N-, or S-containing compounds that are metabolized to species that are deficient, or potentially deficient, in an electron pair; (b) free radicals, which are species that contain an odd number of electrons and may possess a positive, a negative, or no charge, and (c) other neutral reactive species, in which two electrons are lost (e.g. carbenes or nitrenes).

The level of oxygen in myocardial tissue rises dramatically during reperfusion, with oxygen providing an alternative source of radical species known as superoxide ($O_2^{\cdot-}$), following its one or two electron reduction. One electron transfer can be catalysed by any of the following enzymes; xanthine oxidase, by haemoproteins such as haemoglobin, NADPH-cytochrome P-450 reductase and cytochrome P-450 [17, 18]. The superoxide anion is also formed by the mitochondrial electron transport chain, redox cycling and auto-oxidation of endogenous molecules [19].

Superoxide is a highly reactive species which readily undergoes a number of metabolic and chemical reactions. Of these, dismutation to $H_2O_2$ is the most common, a reaction which is catalysed by superoxide dismutase; protonation to form the hydroperoxy radical ($HOO^{\cdot}$) is also possible. In cells the two electron reduction of $O_2$ to $H_2O_2$ can be followed by its rapid detoxication by seleno-protein glutathione peroxidase and by catalase to yield $H_2O$ and $O_2$ [20]. Unfortunately, any $H_2O_2$ that evades this defence mechanism can result in the formation of hydroxyl radicals ($HO^{\cdot}$), which can then participate in radical chain reactions, resulting in the formation of further reactive oxygen species, including singlet oxygen $O^{\cdot}$ [21].

With respect to eukaryotic cells, the majority of oxygen activation occurs mainly within the mitochondria, where the respiratory chain utilizes approximately 90% of oxygen, a factor which can be considerably influenced by re-perfusion following an ischaemic attack. The production of hazardous oxygen radicals is believed to account for approximately 1–2% of mitochondrial oxygen consumption [19]. Under normal conditions, the organelle is protected by an elaborate system of antioxidants and radical scavengers; however, electron flow may not be totally efficient and therefore occasional electron leakage can occur, resulting in the formation of $O_2^{\cdot-}$. This diversion of electrons to oxygen is thought to occur at the ubiquinone-cytochrome b region of the respiratory chain [22]. Although scavengers of $O_2^{\cdot-}$ are very active, like the electron flow mentioned above, their efficiency is not complete and therefore the level of the anion radical will tend to vary.

In general terms, $O_2^{\cdot-}$ generation tends to increase as mitochondria approach state 4 respiration (e.g. substrate and oxygen in excess, ADP absent) when all the components of the respiratory chain are mostly reduced [23]. Animal studies also indicate that steady-state concentrations of $O_2^{\cdot-}$ are higher in mitochondria of older animals [24], therefore the susceptibility and extent of myocardial damage resulting from increased oxygen levels is likely to be related to the age of the individual. Also the major intracellular problems relate to the formation of a more reactive species $HOO^{\cdot}$, $HO^{\cdot}$ or $O^{\cdot}$, all of which have very short lives. The chemical properties of these radicals therefore indicate that their initial site of action is likely to be close to the ubiquinone-cytochrome b complex, and the initiation of peroxidative damage to mitochondrial membrane lipids [25].

The present discussion of peroxidative reactions is restricted to their occurrence in association with the mitochondrion. This organelle has a capacity to utilize oxygen at a high rate, contains high concentrations of polyunsaturated fatty acids (e.g. phosphatidylcholine and phosphatidylethanolamine) and peroxidative catalysts (e.g. haem and nonhaem iron). These features render the mitochondrion vulnerable to damage following re-perfusion hence its high susceptibility to peroxidative-induced injuries. It should be stated, however, that the microsomal system, involving the cytochrome P-450 catalytic cycle, can also generate reactive oxygen species, which may also initiate peroxidative reactions within the cells, especially hepatocytes. This system is sensitive to SKF 525-A, a classical inhibitor of cytochrome P-450 mediate of reactions [26].

Recent studies have indicated the presence of a NAD(P)H/$FE^{3+}$/ADP-dependent lipid peroxidation in mitochondria and in submitochondrial particles isolated from beef heart. Once again, this NADH- or NADPH-dependent lipid peroxidation is catalysed by the NADH dehydrogenase of the respiratory chain, at or near the rotenone-sensitive site. This nucleotide action results in the reduction of the ADP-$Fe^{3+}$ complex and a process that provides the potential to initiate lipid peroxidation. However, under normal circumstances this reduction is unlikely because intact mitochondria are impermeable to reduced nicotinamide nucleotides [27–29]. However, increased permeability may result from one or more of the following: initial lipid peroxidation resulting from radical production from another intracellular site within the cell; the activity of electron systems located in the outer membrane, or in the outer face of the inner membrane, or from damage resulting from re-perfusion. These processes could render the inner membrane sufficiently permeable to NAD(P)H to deliver electrons to the NADH-dehydrogenase complex of the respiratory chain, resulting in radical production.

With respect to $O_2^{\cdot-}$ generation in rat heart mitochondria, Nohl [30] in 1988 demonstrated the existence of an active generating system that operates independently of energy-linked respiration, but requires external (cytosolic) NADH. Evidence suggests that the exogenous NADH dehydrogenase can form an active redox complex with molecular oxygen, yielding univalently reduced dioxygen molecules. In contrast to the 'classical sources', $O_2^{\cdot-}$ from the above enzyme system is not released into the mitochondrial matrix and therefore it does not undergo dismutation to $H_2O_2$ by superoxide dismutase [30].

The conversion of $O_2^{\cdot-}$ into more reactive species (e.g. $^{\cdot}OH$) results in the initiation of peroxidative damage. Thus during lipid peroxidation, free radicals interact with polyunsaturated fatty acids to form lipid peroxy radicals (ROO$^{\bullet}$), which then produce lipid hydroperoxide (ROOH). This process results in the propagation of a peroxidative cascade and the consumption of membrane lipid, resulting in increased membrane permeability (organelle or plasma) and/or potential cell death. In hepatocytes, the onset of cell death can be delayed by the detoxification of lipid radicals by glutathione peroxidase and vitamin E, while hydroalkenals can be readily eliminated by glutathione (GSH) conjugation, catalysed by glutathione S-transferase. With respect to cardiac cells, these defence mechanisms may not be as important, so these cells are potentially more susceptible to irreversible damage. Once again, studies on isolated rat hepatocytes indicate that cell death does not occur until the level of reduced (GSH) falls substantially [31].

The peroxidative action on lipids has deleterious consequences with respect to the re-oxygenated cardiac muscle. The extent of lipid peroxidation on the rate of creatine kinase release was dependent on arterial oxygen tension ($pO_2$), when measured by the production of malondialdehyde (MDA) [8].

Thus the peroxidation of cardiac lipids changes sarcolemmal permeability to ions, releases cellular enzymes, depletes cellular thiols (e.g. GSH) including those in proteins, inhibits prostaglandin synthesis, (thus promoting the production of vasoconstrictor thromboxane $A_2$, causes mitochondrial damage (i.e. the promotion of the aging process), and brings about changes in calcium or potassium fluxes [24, 32–34].

It has been shown that many of the above effects could be prevented by exogenous GSH or superoxide dismutase (SOD), using perfused isolated rat hearts. These beneficial effects probably relate to an improvement in the overall oxidation state of cellular GSH (e.g. GSH : GSSG ratio), which is normally reduced by hypoxia. The protection against oxygen-mediated damage during re-oxygenation provided by GSH is likely to be twofold: (a) inactivation of the superoxide anion; and (b) prevention of peroxidation of unsaturated lipids or denaturation of proteins associated with the sarcolemma or endothelium. With respect to mitochondrial function, the protective effect of GSH is linked to increased matrix selenium-dependent glutathione peroxidase activity and the control of mitochondrial permeability to $Ca^{2+}$ during oxygen readmission [26].

Direct measurements of mitochondrial $Ca^{2+}$ movements have shown that iron-induced lipid peroxidation causes a large release of accumulated $Ca^{2+}$ and $K^+$ ions, the latter being secondary to the efflux of $Ca^{2+}$. In contrast, lipid peroxidation induced by $Fe^{3+}$/ascorbate, cumene hydroperoxide or $Fe^{3+}$/gluconate results in a progressive drop in transmembrane electrical potential, which has been attributed to an enhancement of

*Table 1.* Effects of calcium repletion on cardiac cells

| Initial effects | Prolonged effects |
|---|---|
| Excess influx of $Ca^{2+}$ into cells | Loss of $Ca^{2+}$-dependent contractility |
| Depletion of myocardial high-energy phosphate stores | Washout of nucleotide degradation products |
| Uncoupling of respiration from phosphorylation | Tissues disruption and enzyme release |
| Capacity to synthesize ATP irreversibly lost | Swelling of myocytes and endothelial cells |
| Increased mitochondrial $Ca^{2+}$ uptake | Migration of leucocytes into ischaemic myocardium |
| Calcification of mitochondria | Enhanced free radical production and lipid peroxidation |
| Free radical formation | Cell necrosis |

endogenous $Ca^{2+}$ cycling [35]. $Ca^{2+}$ release from isolated mitochondria also occurs due to an increase in the oxidation states of nicotinamide nucleotides, this increase being stimulated by organic hydroperoxide [33].

Alterations in mitochondrial $Ca^{2+}$ movements are therefore clearly identified as a consequence of lipid peroxidation following oxygen free radical production. It is therefore likely that re-perfusion injury results, in part, from a burst of free radical production during re-oxygenation following the autoxidation of reduced substrates accumulated during ischaemia [36, 37]. These alterations caused by ischaemia-reperfusion markedly affect mitochondrial functions, including respiratory capacity, oxidative phosphorylation and $Ca^{2+}$ movements [38]. Thus, reperfusion causes excessive influx of $Ca^{2+}$ into cardiac cells, which in turn results in the following consequences: depletion of myocardial high-energy phosphate stores; uncoupling of respiration from phosphorylation; irreversible loss in the capacity to synthesize ATP, and irreversible organelle damage. Perfusion and freeze clamping techniques have confirmed that changes in adenine nucleotide and creatine phosphate levels occur within seconds of reoxygenation and $Ca^{2+}$ repletion [39, 40]. Table 1 outlines the initial intracellular changes plus the related effects resulting from re-oxygenation and $Ca^{2+}$ repletion.

In addition to the effects discussed above, increased cytosolic $Ca^{2+}$ levels can lead to onset of cytotoxicity that is not totally linked to changes

*Table 2.* Effect of increased cytosolic calcium levels on key enzymes

| Enzyme | Effect | Site of action | Products |
|---|---|---|---|
| Phospholipase $A_2$ | Activation | Hydrolysis of membrane phospholipids | Lysophospho-lipids, arachidonic acid |
| Proteases | Activation | Cleavage of cytoskeletal or other proteins | Peptide fragments |
| Endonucleases | Activation | DNA strand breaks | Oligo-nucleosone fragments |

in mitochondrial dysfunction, but also relates changes in the activity of $Ca^{2+}$-dependent degradative enzymes, including phospholipases, proteases and endonucleases [7, 41]. Prolonged activation of these enzyme systems resulting in extensive catabolism of cellular constituents and cell death (table 2). With respect to $Ca^{2+}$ overload and resultant myocardial damage, this may be reduced and oxidative phosphorylation maintained by administration of $Ca^{2+}$ antagonists [42–44]. Studies with the $Ca^{2+}$ antagonist nitrendipine and the endogenous acyl carnitine palmitoyl carnitine have shown that these compounds have the ability to alter $Ca^{2+}$ transport into cardiac mitochondria by promoting the release of the ion from the organelle; this effect occurred at concentrations that did not prevent ATP synthesis [45, 46].

Thus, oxygen readmission and $Ca^{2+}$ repletion to the hypoxic myocardium results in the onset of rapid and irreversible toxic effects that can eventually result in the death of cardiac cells. Although a number of organelles or cell components may be involved in the overall process of necrosis, it is likely that mitochondrial related processes are of prime importance for the onset of myocardial cell dysfunction. This is confirmed by the fact that sudden cellular injuries that are triggered by oxygen readmission are dependent upon oxygen tension and re-oxygenation of the mitochondrial electron transfer chain.

## *References*


1 Alpert JS: The pathophysiology of acute myocardial infarction. Cardiology 1989;76:85–95.

2 Wollenberger A, Krause EG: Metabolic control characteristics of acutely ischaemic myocardium. Am J Cardiol 1968;22:349–359.

3 Gudbjarnason S, Mathes P, Ravens KG: Functional compartmentalization of ATP and creatine phosphate in heart muscle. J Mol Cell Cardiol 1970;1:325–329.

4 Braasch W, Gudbjarnason S, Puri PS: Early changes in energy metabolism in the myocardium following acute coronary artery occlusion in anesthetized dogs. Circ Res 1986;23:429–438.

5 Tennant R, Wiggers CJ: The effect of coronary occlusion on myocardial contraction. Am J Physiol 1935;112:351–361.
6 Tennant R: Factors concerned in the arrest of contraction in an ischaemic myocardial area. Am J Physiol 1935;113:677–682.
7 Orrenius S, McConkey DJ, Bellomo G, Nicotera P: Role of $Ca^{2+}$ in toxic cell killing. Trends Pharmacol Sci 1989;10:281–285.
8 Gauduel Y, Menasche P, Duvelleroy M: Enzyme release and mitochondrial activity in reoxygenated cardiac muscle: Relationship with oxygen-induced lipid peroxidation. Gen Physiol Biophys 1989;8:327–340.
9 Bridges JW, Benford DJ, Hubbard SA: Mechanisms of toxic injury. Ann NY Acad Sci 1983;407:42–63.
10 Reimer KA, Jennings R, Tatum AH: Pathobiology of acute myocardial ischaemia: Metabolic, functional and ultrastructural studies. Am J Cardiol 1983;52:72A–80A.
11 Puri PS: Contractile and biochemical effects of coronary reperfusion after extended periods of coronary occlusion. Am J Cardiol 1975;36:244–251.
12 Jennings RB, Schaper J, Hill ML: Effects of reperfusion late in the phase of reversible ischaemic injury. Circ Res 1985;56:262.
13 Braunwald E, Kloner RA: The stunned myocardium: Prolonged post-ischaemic ventricular dysfunction. Circulation 1982;66:1150–1153.
14 Zucci R, Limbruno U, DiVencenzo A, Mariani M, Ronca G: Adenine nucleotide depletion and contractile dysfunction in the 'stunned' myocardium. Cardiol Res 1990;24:440–446.
15 Opie LH: Products of myocardial ischaemia and electrical instability of the heart. J Am Coll Cardiol 1985;5:162B–165B.
16 Hearse DJ, Humphrey SM, Chain EB: Abrupt reoxygenation of the anoxic potassium-arrested perfused rat heart: A study of myocardial enzyme release. J Mol Cell Cardiol 1973;5:395–407.
17 Boobis AR, Fawthrop DJ, Davies DS: Mechanisms of cell death. Trends Pharmacol Sci 1989;10:275–280.
18 Vlessis AA, Mela-Riker L: Potential role of mitochondrial calcium metabolism during reperfusion injury. Am J Physiol 1989;256:1196–1206.
19 Hruszkewycz AM, Bergtold DS: Oxygen radicals, lipid peroxidation and DNA damage in mitochondria. Basic Life Sci 1988;49:449–456.
20 Nohl H: Oxygen radical release in mitochondria: Influence of age; in Johnson JE Jr, Walford R, Harman D, Miguel J (eds): Free Radicals, Aging and Degenerative Diseases. New York, Liss, 1986; pp 77–97.
21 Bindoli A: Lipid peroxidation in mitochondria. Free Radic Biol Med 1988;5:247–261.
22 Nohl H, Jordan W: The mitochondrial site of superoxide formation. Biochem Biophys Res Commun 1986;138:533.
23 Forman HJ, Boveris A: Superoxide radical and hydrogen peroxide in mitochondria; in Pryor WA (ed): Free Radicals in Biology. New York, Academic Press, 1982; vol 5, pp 65–90.
24 Miguel J, Fleming J: Theoretical and experimental support for an 'oxygen radical-mitochondrial injury', hypothesis of cell aging; in Johnson JE Jr, Walford R, Harman D, Miguel J (eds): Free Radicals, Aging and Degenerative Diseases. New York, Liss, 1986.
25 Naqui A, Chance B: Reactive oxygen intermediates in biochemistry. Annu Rev Biochem 1986;55:137–165.
26 Bindoli A: Lipid peroxidation in mitochondria. Free Radic Biol Med 1988;5:247–261.
27 Lehninger AL: Phosphorylation coupled to oxidation of dihydrodiphosphopyridine nucleotide. J Biol Chem 1951;190:345–359.

28 Takayange R, Takeshige K, Minakami S: NADH- and NADPH-dependent lipid peroxidation in bovine heart submitochondrial particles. Biochem J 1980;192:853–860.
29 Takeshige K, Takaganagi R, Minakami S: Lipid peroxidation and the reduction of ADP-$Fe^{3+}$ chelate by NADH-ubiquinone reductase preparation from bovine heart mitochondria. Biochem J 1980;192:861–866.
30 Nohl H: Superoxide radical release into the cytoplasm of heart cells by an NADH-driven oxygen activator. Basic Life Sci 1988;49:899–903.
31 Ekloew-Laoast L, Rossi L, Thor H, Orrenius S: Effects of oxidative stress caused by hypoxia and diquat. A study in isolated hepatocytes. Free Radic Res Commun 1986;2:57–68.
32 Rossi L, Moore GA, Orrenius S, O'Brien PJ: Quinone toxicity in hepatocytes without oxidative stress. Arch Biochem Biophys 1986;251:25–35.
33 Richter C, Frei B: Movements induced by hydroperoxides in mitochondria; in Sies H (ed): Oxidative Stress. London, Academic Press, 1985, pp 221–241.
34 Nohl H, Hegner D: Do mitochondria produce oxygen radicals in vivo? Eur J Biochem 1978;82:563–567.
35 Masini A, Trenti T, Ceccarelli-Stanzani D, Ventura E: The effect of ferric iron complex on isolated rat liver mitochondria. II. Ion movements. Biochim Biophys Acta 1985;810:27–32.
36 Hearse DJ, Humphrey SM, Chain EB: Abrupt reoxygenation of the anoxic potassium-arrested perfused rat heart. A study of myocardium enzyme release. J Mol Cell Cardiol 1973;5:395–407.
37 McCord JM: Superoxide radical: A likely link between reperfusion injury and inflammation. Adv Free Radic Biol Med 1986;2:325–345.
38 Piper HM, Sezer O, Schleyer M, Schwartz P, Hutter JF, Spieckermann PG: Development of ischaemia-induced damage in defined mitochondrial subpopulation. J Mol Cell Cardiol 1985;17:885–896.
39 Unitt JF, McCormick JG, Reid D, MacLachlan LK, England PJ: Direct evidence for a role of intra-mitochondrial $Ca^{2+}$ in the regulation of oxidative phosphorylation in the stimulated rat heart. Biochem J 1989;262:293–301.
40 Zucci R, Limbruno U, DiVincenzo A, Manani M, Ronca G: Adenine nucleotide depletion and contractile dysfunction in the 'stunned' myocardium. Cardiol Res 1990;24:440–446.
41 Nicotera P, McConkey DJ, Dypbukt JM, Jones DP, Orrenius S: $Ca^{2+}$ activated mechanisms in cell killing. Drug Metab Rev 1989;20:193–201.
42 Fleckenstein A: Calcium Antagonists in Heart and Smooth Muscle. New York, Wiley, 1983.
43 Baydoun AR, Markham A, Morgan RM, Sweetman AJ: Modifier of calcium transport and energy metabolism in rat heart mitochondria: A new intracellular site of action. Br J Pharmacol 1990;101:15–20.
44 Markham A, Morgan RM, Sweetman AJ: Determination of the extent of ischaemic damage and the effect of the calcium antagonist verapamil following coronary artery ligation in rat. Methods Find Exp Clin Pharmacol 1990;12:467–472.
45 Watts J, Maiorano P, Harwell T: Comparison of the effects of bepridil and diltiazem upon globally ischaemic rat heart. Eur J Pharmacol 1987;134:25–33.
46 Baydoun AR, Markham A, Morgan RM, Sweetman AJ: Palmitoyl carnitine: An endogenous promoter of calcium efflux from rat heart mitochondria. Biochem Pharmacol 1988;37:3103–3107.

A. Markham, MD, School of Health Sciences, University of Sunderland,
Sunderland SR1 3SD (UK)

Weetman DF, Wood D (eds): Risk Factors for Cardiovascular Disease in Non-Smokers. Int. Workshop, Washington, Tyne and Wear, 1991. Basel, Karger, 1993, pp 33–42

# Development of Arrhythmias in the Ischaemic Heart

*Michael J. Curtis*

Cardiovascular Research Laboratories, Pharmacology Group, King's College, London, UK

Other contributions have considered factors which determine whether or not atherosclerosis and thrombosis occur. In this contribution we shall assume that coronary artery obstruction is present and will analyse the factors which determine whether or not this leads to the production of ventricular arrhythmias. We shall consider briefly the natural history of arrhythmogenesis in the ischaemic heart, and the types of arrhythmias which occur, and discuss in some depth the factors which may determine the severity of arrhythmias associated with ischaemic heart disease.

## *Natural History of Arrhythmogenesis in the Ischaemic Heart*

It is difficult to obtain in man a very precise picture for the time course of development of arrhythmogenesis in early ischaemic heart disease, despite studies such as those of Campbell et al. [1]. Since the first sign of ischaemic heart disease is very often death, it is possible to infer that the interval between the onset of ischaemia and the onset of arrhythmias may be very brief. Although not proven in man, the data from experiments performed in laboratory animals strongly support this viewpoint [2].

Figure 1 shows the natural history of arrhythmogenesis in animal models of ischaemic heart disease, based on data from Curtis et al. [2] and Meesman [3]. There are two main phases: phase I and phase II. In dogs, but not in some other species such as rat, we see two components of phase I, so-called phase Ia and Ib. After a period of 30 min or so, phase I arrhythmias wane, there is a period of quiescence and then phase II commences approximately 90 min after the onset of ischaemia. Insufficient data are available, particularly during the first hour of ischaemia, to indicate whether the same pattern is seen in man as in laboratory animals, but this may well be the case.

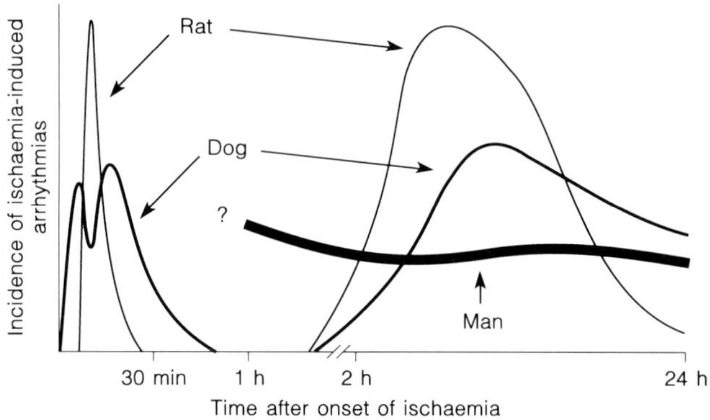


*Fig. 1.* Relationship between duration of ischaemia and incidence of ventricular arrhythmias. The relationship for man is poorly defined; little data exist for less than 1 h after onset of ischaemia. The data are drawn from the literature since 1887.

## *Types of Arrhythmias in Early Myocardial Ischaemia*

Again, information on the types of arrhythmias is almost exclusively derived from animal experiments. In phase I of arrhythmogenesis we see serious ventricular arrhythmias, including premature beats, tachycardia and fibrillation. (These subclasses of ventricular arrhythmias have been defined according to the recent Lambeth Conventions [4].) Fibrillation is the most dangerous (lethal) ventricular arrhythmia, because no coordinated contraction occurs in the ventricle, and within a few minutes death ensues. In phase II, characteristically we see serious ventricular arrhythmias again, but the susceptibility to ventricular fibrillation is not as great as during phase I [2]. As infarction develops, atrial arrhythmias are seen, associated with disturbances in general haemodynamics.

## *Factors Which Determine the Severity of Arrhythmias in the Ischaemic Heart*

Once again we are reliant on data from animal experiments, supported by observations in man. Factors which are likely to be important in determining susceptibility to arrhythmias range from the size and depth of the ischaemic zone through to the more controversial area of stress, and we shall consider each factor in turn.

One would expect to see a relationship between the size of the ischaemic zone and the severity of arrhythmias, and indeed this has been shown very clearly in experiments performed in dogs [5] and in rats [2]. Recently, experiments with rat hearts in my laboratory [6] have shown that the peak of susceptibility to arrhythmias is associated with a condition where roughly equal amounts of ischaemic and nonischaemic tissue exist. This allows speculation about the mechanisms of arrhythmogenesis [7] which will not be explored here, but one can certainly see a very well-defined relationship between ischaemic zone size and incidence of arrhythmia.

Given an ischaemic zone of a particular size, the depth of ischaemia within that zone is an important determinant of susceptibility to arrhythmias. The most important point to note here is that the depth of ischaemia will be determined by the extent and nature of collateral vessels (vessels, other than the main occluded vessel, which can bring blood into the jeopardized region). Indeed, it has been shown that in rats, which have a very low level of residual flow [8], there is a very high susceptibility to arrhythmias [2]. In dogs we see a variable collateral flow: some animals have large levels of collateral flow, others have very little. This has allowed study, within a single species, of the relationship between collateral flow and arrhythmogenesis. Meesmann [3] has extensively analysed this and has shown that in dogs with collaterals, only 1 out of 27 developed ventricular fibrillation following left circumflex occlusion. However, in dogs with no collaterals, 19 out of 19 developed ventricular fibrillation.

The dependence on collateral flow is very clear. This suggests an interesting hypothesis, that as we age, and our coronary vessels show pathological changes, this stimulates the development of collaterals. Paradoxically, it may be that as we age the likelihood of ischaemic heart disease increases, but the likelihood of this producing ventricular fibrillation may decline: there are many anecdotes of relatively young, supposedly fit and healthy people who die suddenly of ventricular fibrillation. Perhaps these are people who have not yet developed collateral vessels.

The next factor to consider is the occurrence of reperfusion. Clinically, ischaemia may be transient and self-limiting, associated with either relief of vasospasm or spontaneous thrombolysis. Reversal of ischaemia results in reperfusion, and it has been shown in animal experiments that reperfusion is an extremely potent arrhythmogenic stimulus [2]. There is little data on this in man, apart from a much quoted case report from Tzivoni et al. [9] which showed relief of vasospasm precipitating ventricular fibrillation.

What is the natural history of reperfusion arrhythmias? We have found a bell-shaped relationship between susceptibility to reperfusion-induced ventricular fibrillation and the duration of preceding ischaemia in isolated rat heart [10]. With very brief durations of ischaemia (5–10 min) reperfusion of the tissues gave a high incidence of ventricular fibrillation (up to 100% incidence), but this susceptibility declines quite rapidly with longer durations of ischaemia. This implies that perhaps in variant angina, which is characterized by brief episodes of ischaemia, we are likely to encounter reperfusion-induced ventricular fibrillation. Many clinicians would argue that reperfusion is not an important factor in sudden cardiac death due to ventricular fibrillation. One reason for this apparent disagreement may be that clinicians often see patients reperfused, especially those electively reperfused, after a long maintained period of ischaemia: in these circumstances one would not expect to see a high susceptibility to ventricular fibrillation (if the bell-shaped relationship applies to man). Another explanation is based on consideration of results from animal experiments which show that repeated episodes of ischaemia cause a phenomenon called preconditioning, whereby the susceptibility of the heart to reperfusion injury, including ventricular fibrillation, is reduced [11]. Thus, it may be that clinicians commonly see patients with preconditioned myocardia, unpreconditioned patients having died of their first transient ischaemia attack.

It has been shown that in man there is a strong inverse relationship between cardiovascular mortality and blood potassium concentration [12]. Animal experiments have also shown clearly that blood potassium levels influence susceptibility to ischaemia-induced ventricular fibrillation. For instance, figure 2 shows results from conscious rats in which blood potassium levels were modified by various manipulations and the incidence of ischaemia-induced ventricular fibrillation was plotted against the range of blood potassium concentrations for the various sub-groups [13]. We can see that as blood potassium concentration increased, susceptibility to ventricular fibrillation declined markedly, so that with relatively high blood potassium concentrations relatively few animals developed ventricular fibrillation. Additional experiments have shown that this effect of potassium is mediated within the uninvolved tissue and is not related to changes within the ischaemic zone [10]. Undoubtedly there are changes in potassium homeostasis in the ischaemic zone, but these are not the basis for the antiarrhythmic effects of high blood potassium. It is important to note that this effect of potassium is one of the few unequivocal examples where a procedure which modulates ventricular fibrillation in animal models of ischaemic heart disease equates with a risk factor for cardiovascular mortality in man in every case for which this has been examined. There are other factors for which attempts have been made to relate animal data to clinical data, but with mixed results: in the case of potassium the results are always in agreement [13].

Other contributors have dealt with lipids and phospholipids as determinants of the occurrence of atherogenesis and ischaemia. There is not a great deal of data on these substances when considering the occurrence of

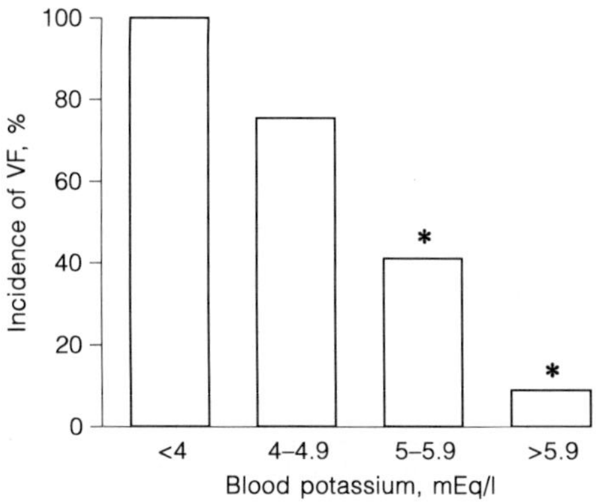


*Fig. 2.* Relationship between blood potassium concentration and incidence of phase 1 ischaemia-induced ventricular fibrillation (VF) in conscious rats. $^{*}p < 0.05$ vs. $< 4$ mEq/l potassium. Data from Curtis et al. [13].

arrhythmias once ischaemia is established. However, studies such as that of McLennan et al. [14] do suggest some relationship between incidence of ischaemia-induced arrhythmias in rats and the dietary lipid content.

The study of Pocock et al. [15] demonstrated a strong relationship between susceptibility to cardiovascular mortality and the electrolyte content of drinking water, particularly with calcium and nitrate levels. The calcium data (high levels apparently protective) are rather difficult to explain and it may be that the relationship between calcium and cardiovascular mortality is casual rather than causal. Recently we have looked at nitrate, and we were surprised to find that the relationship in humans seems to be supported by experiments on ventricular fibrillation and extracellular anion content in the isolated heart [16, 17]. We found that replacement of chloride with anions with differing membrane permeabilities determined the likelihood of ventricular fibrillation [18]. Figure 3 shows data from experiments in isolated rat heart where the incidence of ischaemia-induced ventricular fibrillation was studied whilst the major anion in the Krebs-bicarbonate solution was altered [18]. We see remarkable differences in the incidence of ventricular fibrillation with different anions and the rank order of incidence of ventricular fibrillation correlates with the rank order of membrane permeability for these particular anions: introduction of the highly permeant ions nitrate or iodide reduced the incidence of fibrillation to zero. These findings are under further study.

The last factor, and perhaps the most difficult one to consider, is stress. The word 'stress' is difficult to define and is used here as a diffuse term covering a variety of factors which can be regarded as being related.

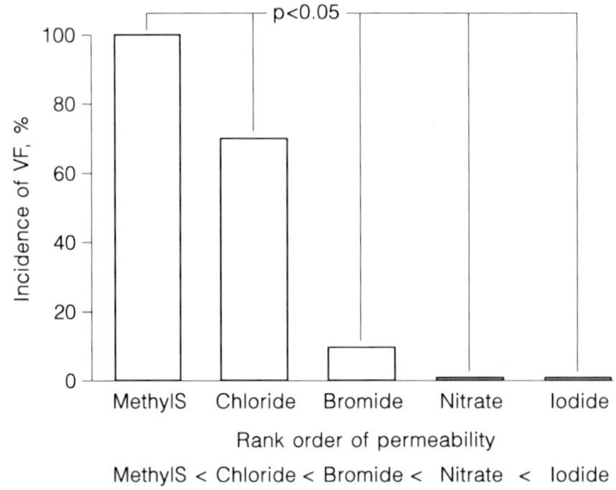


*Fig. 3.* Relationship between identity of major anion in perfusion solution and incidence of phase 1 ischaemia-induced arrhythmias in isolated rat heart. Rank order of permeability corresponds with rank order of effectiveness in suppressing ventricular fibrillation (VF). Data from Ridley et al. [18].

Again, we are not discussing the relationship between stress and the development of ischaemic heart disease, but whether stress influences arrhythmogenesis once occlusion has occurred, so again there is not a great deal of data available. The effects of antisympathetic drugs or of ablation of the sympathetic nervous system on development of arrhythmias have been examined and the results indicate that on balance the level of the sympathetic nervous input to the heart does not appear to have a great influence on susceptibility to ischaemia-induced ventricular fibrillation [13, 19]. There is quite a lot of data which suggests that the sympathetic nervous system determines whether or not ventricular fibrillation occurs in ischaemic heart disease [e.g. 20], but also a huge amount of data which suggests that it is not very important [13]. However, $\beta$-adrenoceptor tone does appear to influence susceptibility to arrhythmias, but not by a direct effect in the heart: the effect appears to be dependent on the relationship between adrenoceptor tone and blood potassium concentration [13]. This has been demonstrated in several recent studies in animals, all of which indicate that the $\beta_2$-adrenoceptor tone in skeletal muscle affects blood potassium homeostasis and that this has a profound influence on the susceptibility to ischaemia-induced arrhythmias [13].

Heart rate is another factor loosely associated with stress. Heart rate appears to modulate susceptibility to arrhythmogenesis [21], but this seems to be an indirect effect: the onset of ventricular fibrillation appears to be delayed or speeded up depending upon the heart rate, but if the experiment is followed through over a sustained period of 30–40 min, most of the hearts will fibrillate eventually. One can conclude that it is the timing of the onset of arrhythmia which seems to be affected by heart rate rather than whether or not arrhythmias occur.

The last point related to stress can be described as ambient conditions. There is not a great deal of data on this, and it is a little confusing. For instance, it was shown (perhaps surprisingly) that chronic isolation and hypothermia reduced susceptibility to ischaemia-induced arrhythmias in rats [22], but on the other hand, familiarization with housing conditions was shown to reduce arrhythmias induced by coronary occlusion in pigs [20].

In summary, the risk factors for ventricular fibrillation once occlusion has occurred can be ranked in order of perceived importance. I consider the most important factors to be the presence or absence of ischaemia and the size of the ischaemic zone: next, the depth of the ischaemic zone, determined by collateral blood supply. Thirdly, the occurrence of reperfusion is high in priority because reperfusion is such a powerful arrhythmogenic stimulus, and if it does occur after brief periods of ischaemia, there is a very great likelihood that it will induce ventricular fibrillation. Next, blood potassium concentration: a neglected factor and there may be curious and interesting reasons why this is so. Fifth: dietary lipids and electrolyte content of drinking water: the data here are not so strong or are rather new and unsubstantiated. The last point I would list is stress.

## *References*


1 Campbell RWF, Murray A, Julian DG: Ventricular arrhythmias in the first 12 hours after acute myocardial infarction: Natural history study. Br Heart J 1981;46:351–357.

2 Curtis MJ, Macleod BA, Walker MJA: Models for the study of arrhythmias in myocardial ischemia and infarction: The use of the rat. J Mol Cell Cardiol 1987;19:399–419.

3 Meesman W: Early arrhythmias and primary ventricular fibrillation after acute myocardial ischemia in relation to pre-existing coronary collaterals; in Parratt JR (ed): Early Arrhythmias Resulting from Myocardial Ischemia. London, Macmillan, 1982, pp 139–151.

4 Walker MJA, Curtis MJ, Hearse DJ, Campbell RFW, Janse MJ, Yellon DM, Cobbe SM, Coker SJ, Harness JB, Harron DWG: The Lambeth Conventions: Guidelines for the study of arrhythmias in ischaemia, infarction and reperfusion. Cardiovasc Res 1988;22;447–455.

5 Austin M, Wenger TL, Harrell FE, Luzzi FA, Strauss HC: Effect of myocardium at risk on outcome after coronary occlusion and release. Am J Physiol 1982;243:H340–H345.

6 Ridley PD, Yacoub MH, Curtis MJ: A modified model of global ischaemia: Application to the study of syncytial mechanisms of arrhythmogenesis. Cardiovasc Res 1992;26:313–322.

7 Curtis MJ, Hearse DJ: Reperfusion-induced arrhythmias are critically dependent on occluded zone size: Relevance to the mechanism of arrhythmogenesis. J Mol Cell Cardiol 1989;21:625–637.

8 Maxwell MP, Hearse DJ, Yellon DM: Species variation in the coronary collateral circulation during regional myocardial ischemia: A critical determinant of the rate of evolution and extent of myocardial infarction. Cardiovasc Res 1987;21:737–746.

9 Tzivoni D, Keren A, Granot H, Gottlieb S, Benhorin J, Stern A: Ventricular fibrillation caused by myocardial perfusion in Prinzmetal's angina. Am Heart J 1983;105:323–325.

10 Curtis MJ, Hearse DJ: Ischemia-induced and reperfusion-induced arrhythmias differ in their sensitivity to potassium: Implications for the mechanism of initiation versus the mechanism of maintenance of ventricular fibrillation. J Mol Cell Cardiol 1989;21:21–40.

11 Shiki K, Hearse DJ: Preconditioning of the ishemic myocardium: Reperfusion-induced arrhythmias. Am J Physiol 1987;253:H1470–H1476.

12 Nordrehaug JE, Von Der Lippe G: Hypokalemia and vertricular fibrillation in acute myocardial infarction. Br Heart J 1983;50:525–529.

13 Curtis MJ, Botting JH, Hearse DJ, Walker MJA: The sympathetic nervous system, catecholamines and ischaemia-induced arrhythmias: Dependence upon serum potassium concentration; in Brachman J, Schomig A (eds): Adrenergic System and Ventricular Arrhythmias in Myocardial Infarction. Berlin, Springer, 1989, pp 205–219.

14 McLennan PL, Abeywardena MY, Charnock JS: Influence of dietary lipids on arrhythmias and infarction after coronary artery ligation in rats. Can J Physiol Pharmacol 1985;63:1411–1417.

15 Pocock SJ, Shaper AG, Cook DG, Packham RF, Lacey RF, Powel P, Russell PF: British Regional Heart Study: Geographic variations in cardiovascular mortality, and the role of water quality. Br Med J 1980;280:1243–1249.

16 Ridley PD, Curtis MJ: Nitrates and drinking water: Relationship to cardiac death. Eur Heart J 1990;11:1135–1136.

17 Ridley PD: Anion manipulation, a new antiarrhythmic approach: Action of substitution of chloride with nitrate on ischemia- and reperfusion-induced ventricular fibrillation and contractile function. Circ Res 1992;70:617–632.

18 Ridley PD, Yacoub MH, Curtis MJ: Membrane permeability is a determinant of arrhythmogenesis following anion substitution. Br J Pharmacol 1990;101:511P.

19 Bolli R, Fisher DJ, Tayler AA, Young JB, Miller RR: Effect of alpha-adrenergic blockade on arrhythmias induced by acute myocardial ischemia and reperfusion in the dog. J Mol Cell Cardiol 1984;16:1101–1117.

20 Skinner JE, Lie JT, Entman ML: Modification of ventricular fibrillation latency following coronary artery occlusion in the conscious pig: The effects of psychological stress and beta-adrenergic blockade. Circulation 1975;51:656–667.

21 Bernier M, Curtis MJ, Hearse DJ: Ischemia-induced and reperfusion-induced arrhythmias: Importance of heart rate. Am J Physiol 1989;256:H21–H31.

22 Harris N, Kane KA, Muir AW, Winslow E: Influence of hypothermia, cold and isolation stress on the severity of coronary artery ligation-induced arrhythmias in rats. J Pharmacol Methods 1982;7:161–171.


Dr. Michael J. Curtis, Cardiovascular Research Laboratories, Pharmcology Group, Kings College, Manresa Road, London SW3 6LX (UK)

## *Discussion*

*Roe* (Wimbledon): You seem to be suggesting that high plasma potassium is a protective factor: in my early experience as a houseman this wasn't my impression. Firstly a patient receiving three different sources of potassium developed severe bradycardia and subsequently died; secondly, sudden death was not uncommon amongst patients receiving potassium citrate following prostatectomy; and thirdly the cardiologists noted ECG disturbances and occasional death following injections of potassium.

*Curtis* (London): I am basing my comments on many studies and it's difficult to comment on a couple of anecdotes. First of all, one would need to see exactly what the blood potassium levels were in these patients: clearly there's a bell-shaped relationship with many interventions and you can move out of the beneficial range, so it's rather difficult to explain this without further information.

*Lorimer* (Glasgow): In the context of coronary care it was the initial impression that the use of streptokinase as a thrombolytic agent was leading to an increased incidence of reperfusion arrhythmias, especially ventricular fibrillation. There have however been several studies now published suggesting that the incidence of ventricular fibrillation following reperfusion is not greater than previously. The second point is with regard to potassium: I agree with you it's important but it was always suggested that one of the problems with the thiazide diuretics in high blood pressure would be that there would be hypokalaemia and that this might lead to an increased incidence of sudden death. Certainly this has not been particularly well substantiated, even with some studies looking at potassium in detail. I wonder if you could comment on both of these?

*Curtis:* Let's start with the second part first. Obviously it depends upon how low you bring the blood potassium, and it depends whether you've got ischaemic heart disease too, and it may simply be a case of having to filter out all the noise from the signal in the analysis. To go to the first point, as I tried to show, whether or not you get reperfusion-induced ventricular arrhythmias, fibrillation in particular, is critically dependent upon when you reperfuse, and of course in human beings elective reperfusion tends to occur perhaps several hours at the very earliest after the onset of ischaemia, and if humans are anything like animals then they are not likely to be terribly susceptible to reperfusion-induced arrhythmias at this time. I would say if you electively reperfuse someone and they go into ventricular fibrillation you should feel very happy, because it shows you've reperfused and the tissue is alive.

*Sneddon* (Sunderland): I was interested in your observations on nitrates..Is this another function for EDRF (endothelium-derived relaxant factor), to use its major metabolite as a coronary protective agent, rather than the EDRF itself?

*Curtis:* I am not sure, since I haven't done any work on EDRF although we are planning some. Another aspect of EDRF is its property to be an antiradical agent, and one wonders whether nitric oxide may serve as an endogenous protective agent. We're wondering that if we block EDRF production this might promote reperfusion arrhythmias which are regarded as being dependent in part on the production of oxyradicals.

*Sneddon:* It has been claimed that the epithelial cell is a major source of blood nitrate. If you inhibit EDRF production in the whole animal with NG-nitro-*L*-arginine methyl ester then the urinary nitrate output drops to practically zero so in a normal animal the nitrate appears to be derived from EDRF or nitric oxide.

*Werko* (Göteborg): What about another ion, magnesium?

*Curtis:* Yes, there's a lot of interest in magnesium. Magnesium has been reported to be antiarrhythmic in ischaemia and reperfusion in various models; Crampton and Clark [Circulation 1983;68(suppl 111):146] and Woodward and Zakaria [J Physiol 1983;343:55P–

56P] have done some work on this although I haven't myself. Lots of claims have been made, about magnesium being nature's endogenous calcium antagonist for example. Certainly in the heart that's not likely since according to Beeler and Reuter [J Physiol 1970;207:191–209] you need a concentration of 10 m*M* to block the slow inward currents. It does seem that there's something there, all the reports are positive but I don't know what the mechanism is.

# Intrinsic Factors

Weetman DF, Wood D (eds): Risk Factors for Cardiovascular Disease in Non-Smokers.
Int. Workshop, Washington, Tyne and Wear, 1991. Basel, Karger, 1993, pp 43–49

## Cardiovascular Risk Factors: Heredity and Gender

*R.S. Houlston*

Department of Clinical Genetics, Royal Free Hospital School of Medicine, London, UK

The past 50 years have seen changing patterns in the incidence of cardiovascular disease which have not been confined to any one age group [1], thus supporting the importance of environmental influences on cardiovascular risk.

At first sight a substantial genetic basis to cardiovascular disease would therefore seem unlikely. However, a major role for genetic factors in determining cardiovascular risk has come about with the recognition that the known risk factors cannot entirely account for the development of cardiovascular disease in individuals. Furthermore, it is clear that a large component of the known risk factors is directly attributable to genetic variation. The risks of cardiovascular disease have been shown to be consistently greater for men than women; the disparity is greatest below age 55 when the risk of coronary heart disease in men is approximately six-fold greater than for women. This sex difference has been shown in a number of countries (table 1) and whilst there may be some differences in lifestyle, the principal difference between the sexes is clearly a genetic one.

### *Inheritance of Liability to Cardiovascular Disease*

Direct evidence for the role of genetic factors in determining cardiovascular disease comes from the study of twins and studies of familial aggregation.

#### *Twin Studies*

Comparisons of the concordance rates (similarity) for cardiovascular disease between monozygotic (identical) twins and dizygotic (non-identical) twins have supported the role of genetic factors in cardiovascular disease. Monozygotic twins show higher concordance rates than dizygotic twins of

*Table 1.* Coronary heart disease mortality ratios in selected countries, 1977 [data adapted from 12]

| Country | Male/female ratio age 35–74 |
|---|---|
| Norway | 3.44 |
| Finland | 3.30 |
| USA | 2.56 |
| Scotland | 2.50 |
| Japan | 2.06 |
| Israel | 1.82 |

*Table 2.* Concordative rates for coronary heart disease in twins

| Author(s) | Sex | | Zygosity | Concordance ratios | |
|---|---|---|---|---|---|
| Harvald and Harge, 1970 [13] | M.M. | | MZ | 0.39 | |
| | | | DZ | 0.26 | |
| | F.F. | | MZ | 0.44 | |
| | | | DZ | 0.14 | |
| | F.M. | | DZ, male probands | 0.13 | |
| | | | DZ, female probands | 0.43 | |
| de Faire, 1974 [14] | M.M. | 46 to 70-year-olds | MZ | 0.90 | |
| | | | DZ | 0.62 | |
| | F.F. | | MZ | 1.00 | |
| | | | DZ | 0.89 | |
| Berg, 1981 [15] | Sex-matched | | MZ | 0.65 | |
| | | | DZ | 0.25 | |
| | | | MZ | 0.83 | CHD < 60 |
| | | | DZ | 0.21 | CHD < 60 |

the same sex (table 2). However, the difference is greater for female rather than male pairs. Furthermore, the concordance rates are highest among dizygotic pairs if the female twin is the proband (i.e. the index case in studies tracking a disease through a family).

*Table 3.* Risks of coronary heart disease in first-degree relatives of patients with coronary heart disease

| Author(s) | Patients | Relative risk (RR) |
|---|---|---|
| Slack and Evans, 1966 [16] | male proband, male relatives | 2.47 (proband < 55, relatives < 55 RR = 5.16) |
| | male proband, female relatives | 1.93 (proband < 55, relatives < 55 RR = 2.75) |
| | female proband, male relatives | 3.17 (proband < 55, relatives < 55 RR = 6.44) |
| | female proband, female relatives | 2.77 (proband < 55, relatives < 55 RR = 6.92) |
| Rissanen, 1979 [17, 18] | | 3.5 (proband < 55 RR = 11.0) |
| Nora et al., 1980 [2] | | 10.4 (proband < 55)<br>7.1 (proband < 65) |
| Friedlander et al., 1985 [19] | | 2.78 |

*Table 4.* Risk of early onset ischaemic heart disease (IHD), retrospective cases vs. matched controls [data adapted from 2]

| Factor | Risk ratio | p |
|---|---|---|
| IHD – first-degree relative 55 years | 10.4 | <0.001 |
| IHD – first-degree relative 65 years | 7.1 | <0.001 |
| Insulin-dependent diabetes – first-degree relative | 4.7 | <0.05 |
| Cholesterol > 7.0 mmol/l | 4.3 | <0.001 |
| Smoking > 10 cigarettes/day | 4.0 | <0.001 |
| Hypertension | 1.8 | <0.01 |

*Family Studies*

An increased risk of cardiovascular disease has been consistently shown for first-degree relatives (parents and siblings) of patients with cardiovascular disease (table 3). The risk appears to be greatest for those relatives of patients who develop cardiovascular disease at a young age. Family history has also been shown to be the largest of known risk factors (table 4) and the familial aggregation of coronary heart disease has been shown not to be exclusively mediated through familial resemblance in cholesterol levels or other known risk factors [2]. Prospective studies examining the putative strength of a positive family history after adjustment for the known risk factors have supported these studies and have shown that family history appears to be most strongly related to premature coronary heart disease [3, 4].

### *Model of Liability to Cardiovascular Disease*

The majority of the genetic risk in the general population is not attributable to variation at a single gene locus, but is best explained by polygenic inheritance, with variation at a number of different genes, each having a small effect but contributing to the total genetic liability. The total liability to cardiovascular disease is determined by both genetic and environmental factors.

This is conceptualized in figure 1 from the model proposed by Falconer [5] in 1965 in which there is a normal distribution of total liability with a threshold beyond which individuals are affected with cardiovascular disease. If there was no environmental component contributing to cardiovascular disease, the first-degree relatives of those affected would have a mean liability between those affected and the population mean. However, this is not the case and the difference between the observed number of affected first-degree relatives and the expected indicates the extent of the environmental component to the total variation in liability; the proportion of the total liability contributed by genetic factors is called the heritability.

Since women are less affected than men with cardiovascular disease, those affected will be found more to the right of the liability scale and therefore pass on an increased risk to their first-degree relatives.

The molecular basis of the difference in risk seen in the relatives of male and female patients may in part be attributable to a process known as genetic imprinting, which may account for a large proportion of the heterogeneity seen clinically in many diseases. In this process the differential effects of genes are dependent on the sex of the transmitting parent [for review, see 6].

### *Estimates of the Hereditability of Cardiovascular Disease*

The hereditability of early onset coronary heart disease has been estimated from family studies to be around 60% [2]. Genetic-epidemiological studies have estimated that approximately 50% of early coronary heart disease is associated with a strong familial tendency which is present in

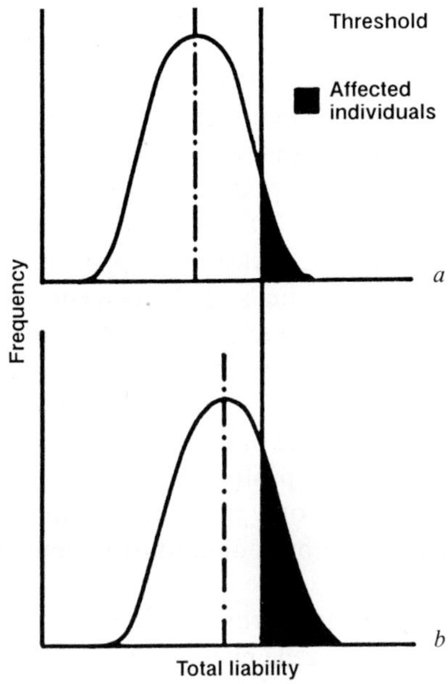


*Fig. 1.* The Falconer model of cardiovascular total liability. *a* Population. *b* First-degree relatives of affected individuals.

only 5–7% of the general population [7]. Some methods of determining estimates of hereditability have not allowed for family resemblance due to common environment, nor the presence of major gene effects, and may have lead to an overestimation of hereditability. Whilst it is unlikely that a shared childhood common environment will play a major role in biasing hereditability, it is recognised that there are some individuals who inherit genes which have a major effect on cardiovascular risk, such as that seen in familial hypercholesterolaemia [for review, see 8].

### *Relevance of the Genetic Influence on Known Risk Factors: Cholesterol Levels*

Epidemiological studies have identified levels of cholesterol, raised blood pressure and cigarette smoking as primary risk factors. Both circulating levels of cholesterol and blood pressure are in part genetically determined.

Interestingly, correlations of cholesterol levels between parent and offspring have shown a higher correlation between mother and offspring than between father and offspring [9], which is reminiscent of the effect seen in overall risks of cardiovascular disease.

Extensive studies suggest that up to 50% of the variability in cholesterol levels in the general population is attributable to genetic differences among individuals [10, 11]. Within this genetic milieu, it is recognised that there is a small number of diseases that have a major effect on cardiovascular disease risk. Familial hypercholesterolaemia is the best described and is caused by a defective gene for the low density lipoprotein (LDL) receptor. LDL particles, which are the major carriers of cholesterol within the circulation, accumulate, and levels exceeding twice the upper range of normal are commonly seen in affected individuals. Fifty percent of men carrying the defective gene will suffer a heart attack by age 50. This risk is ten times that expected for men with cholesterol levels greater than the 95th centile. In contrast, by the age of 50, only 12% of women affected with familial hypercholesterolaemia will have evidence of coronary heart disease. Although familial hypercholesterolaemia has a profound impact on cardiovascular risk, affecting 1 in 500 individuals, it only accounts for about 1 in 20 cases of early coronary heart disease. The bulk of cardiovascular risk is attributable to polygenic variation.

The proportion of genetic liability to cardiovascular disease attributable to polygenes as opposed to single gene effects is of considerable importance. The greater the proportion determined polygenically the greater is the opportunity for reducing disease by environmental manipulations of known risk factors. This is because any environmental change that leads to a decrease in overall liability will cause a significant shift in the number of individuals exceeding the threshold of affection. However, such manipulations will clearly have little impact on those whose risk is principally determined by variation at a single genetic locus.

## *Conclusions*

There is now clear evidence that genetic factors play a major role in mediating the development of cardiovascular risk. Both single genes with a major effect on risk and polygenes contribute to the liability to develop coronary heart disease. The recognition of these different types of inheritance is of considerable importance since those who inherit genes with a major effect need to be identified and rigorously treated, whereas for the majority, whose genetic liability is polygenically determined, a reduction in risk will be achievable by small modifications in the known risk factors. It must be stressed that overzealous modification of any single risk determinate alone will not be productive. There is considerable difference in the risks of cardiovascular disease for men and women and to their offspring; this information should have a bearing on risk management in clinical practice.

## *References*


1 Registrar General's Statistical Reviews of Mortality, England and Wales 1939–1989. London, HMSO, 1989.
2 Nora JJ, Lortscher RH, Spangler RD, Nora AH, Kimberling WJ: Genetic-epidemiologic study of early-onset ischaemic heart disease. Circulation 1980;61:503–506.
3 Sholtz RI, Rosenmann RH, Brand RJ: The relationship of reported parental history to the incidence of coronary heart disease in the Western Collaborative Group Study. Am J Epidemiol 1975;102:350–356.
4 ten Kate LP, Boman H, Daiger SP, Motulsky AG: Familial aggregation of heart disease and its relation to known risk factors. Am J Cardiol 1982;50:945–953.
5 Falconer DS: The inheritance of liability to certain diseases, estimated from the incidence among relatives. Ann Hum Genet 1965;29:51–76.
6 Sapienza C: Parental imprinting of genes. Sci Am 1990;263:26–32.
7 Williams RR: Population-based perspectives of the genetic epidemiology of early coronary disease in Framingham and Utah; in Genetic Epidemiology of Coronary Heart Disease: Past, Present, Future. New York, Liss, 1984, pp 89–91.
8 Brown MS, Goldstein JL: How LDL receptors influence cholesterol and atherosclerosis. Sci Am 1984;251:52–60.
9 Adlersberg D, Schaefer LE, Steinberg AS: Studies on genetic and environmental control of serum cholesterol level. Circulation 1957;16:487–488.
10 Rao DC, Morton NE, Gulbrandsen CL, Rhoads GG, Kagan A, Yee S: Cultural and biological determinants of lipoprotein concentrations. Ann Hum Genet 1979;42:467–477.
11 Moll PP, Powsner R, Sing CF: Analysis of genetic and environmental source of variation in serum cholesterol in Techumseh, Michigan vs. variance components estimated from pedigrees. Ann Hum Genet 1979;42:343–354.
12 Goldbourt U, Neufeld HN: Genetic aspects of arteriosclerosis. Arteriosclerosis 1986;6:357–377.
13 Harvald B, Harge M: Coronary occlusion in twins. Acta Genet Med Gemell, 1970;19:248–250.
14 de Faire U: Ischaemic heart disease in death of discordant twins. A study of 205 male and female pairs. Acta Med Scand 1974;(suppl 568):5–109.
15 Berg K: Twin research in coronary heart disease; in Parisi G-L, Nanie WE (eds): Twin Research 3: Epidemiological and Clinical Studies. New York, Liss, 1981, pp 117–130.
16 Slack J, Evans KA: The increased risk of death from ischaemic heart disease in first-degree relatives of 121 men and 96 women with ischaemic heart disease. J Med Genet 1966;3:239–257.
17 Rissanen A: Familial aggregation of coronary heart disease in a high incidence area (North Karelia, Finland). Br Heart J 1979;42:294–303.
18 Rissanen A: Familial occurrence of coronary heart disease. Effect of age at diagnosis. Am J Cardiol 1979;44:60–66.
19 Friedlander Y, Kark JD, Stein Y: Family history of myocardial infarction as an independent risk factor for coronary heart disease. Br Heart J 1985;53:382–387.


R.S. Houlston, MD MSc MRCPath, Department of Clinical Genetics,
Royal Free Hospital School of Medicine, Pond Street, London NW3 2QG (UK)

Weetman DF, Wood D (eds): Risk Factors for Cardiovascular Disease in Non-Smokers. Int. Workshop, Washington, Tyne and Wear, 1991. Basel, Karger, 1993, pp 50–56

# Impaired Respiratory Function (Reduced $FEV_1$)

*Austin J.S. Gardiner*

Monklands District General Hospital, Airdrie, Lanarkshire, UK

I wish to consider the evidence for respiratory impairment as a risk factor for cardiovascular disease, by examining the results of clinical and epidemiological studies. The clinical consequences on the respiratory system of cardiovascular disease are well known, although not often discussed when considering the individual patient and his therapy, the focus usually centring on the heart itself. There is more often a tendency to consider clinical consequences in the reverse situation, i.e. the effects on the heart of pulmonary disease which results in cor pulmonale or pulmonary heart disease.

There is undoubted evidence of an epidemiological relationship between respiratory dysfunction or impairment and risk of other diseases and their outcomes, most pertinently coronary heart disease. Recent work reaffirms observations in this area which were made at least 15 years ago and it is pertinent to re-examine the relationship.

## *Clinical Observations*

The functional integration of the heart with the respiratory system is so close that one often refers to the cardiorespiratory system. Disordered function of one component may produce disordered function of the other. The symptomatic evidence of respiratory dysfunction is, of course, breathlessness. Clinicians try to distinguish between the possible causes of breathlessness by seeking evidence of wheezing, which suggests a respiratory origin. This is by no means a clear-cut distinguishing feature, however, as acute pulmonary oedema consequent on sudden cardiac failure may lead, in a minority of patients, to severe wheezing accompanying their sensation of breathlessness. Breathlessness may be cardiac in origin, as will emerge in subsequent discussion, but is, of course, usual in the common respiratory diseases of asthma and chronic obstructive pulmonary disease (COPD).

The four principal cardiac pathologies encountered in Western medicine are coronary heart disease, pulmonary heart disease, hypertensive heart disease and valvular heart disease. Such has become the preponderance of coronary heart disease in clinical practice that one may be forgiven for forgetting that valvular heart disease, secondary to acute rheumatism, was the form most commonly seen in the late 19th and early 20th century, thereby forming the basis of descriptive clinical cardiology. The commonest result of rheumatic valvular heart disease was disease of the mitral valve, most particularly stenosis. Although in certain clinical circumstances, such as atrial fibrillation during pregnancy, mitral stenosis could lead acutely to pulmonary oedema, more frequently it resulted in chronic pulmonary hypertension.

The pathological consequences of heart disease can be considered as follows. Coronary artery disease may affect pulmonary function acutely or insidiously. A simple mechanical explanation is not difficult to comprehend. If the left ventricular pump cannot deal with the blood returning to its chamber in unit time, then pressure is reflected back from the left atrium, through the pulmonary circulation to the pulmonary capillaries, where Starling relationships are disturbed, so that the normally dry air spaces and lung interstitium become oedematous, stiffer, and therefore less compliant. The individual senses this as breathlessness. Distension of the pulmonary veins leads to pulmonary congestion where a competition for space within the bronchovascular sheath occurs. In cardiac failure of gradual onset, this mechanism precedes the formation of oedema fluid. It also increases lung stiffness and causes breathlessness. The endstage of untreated hypertensive heart disease is akin to coronary heart disease and its respiratory consequences and will cause breathlessness for the same reasons.

When the initial dysfunction of disease arises in the respiratory system (cor pulmonale), the most serious functional consequences is reduction in arterial oxygen tension, i.e. a reduction of oxygen dissolved in plasma. Unlike the systemic arterioles, the pulmonary arterioles are sensitive to oxygen tension and constrict when this falls below normal. Should this situation persist, then, because of increased workload, the right ventricle will dilate and eventually fall. There are several additional and complex mechanisms which contribute to this failure, such as neutrophil polymorphonuclear leucocyte aggregation, polycythaemia and lung water shift.

Respiratory function may be thought of in four ways: the volumes which determine the availability of atmospheric oxygen to blood; the functions of the airways which connect the lungs to the atmosphere and distribute atmospheric air within the lungs; the relationship of circulation to ventilation which results in normal oxygen saturation and blood gas tensions; lastly, the mechanics of the entire system. These parameters may all be measured in patients with cardiac pathologies.

In coronary heart disease, the spectrum runs from the asymptomatic state to myocardial infarction in which there is severe damage to the left ventricle. In terms of respiratory consequences, VC (vital capacity), FEV25–75 (forced expiratory volume between 25 and 75% VC) and $FEV_1$ (FEV in 1 s) are sharply reduced after myocardial infarction. The aforementioned mechanisms of pulmonary congestion and pulmonary oedema alter regional mechanical function. One effect is to increase the closing volume of the lung, thereby reducing lower lobe perfusion and resulting in a fall in oxygen tension. Clinical studies in the 1970s [1] and early 1980s [2] showed that these functional abnormalities persist for several weeks following myocardial infarction. Longer term studies of patients with coronary heart disease have shown that pulmonary hypertension on exercise is common in men who have made an apparently normal recovery from myocardial infarction and probably accounts for exertional dyspnoea in these subjects [3].

In closing my comments on these clinical observations, I should emphasize that these always refer to small groups of individuals in individual studies, and I have enlarged on them in order to examine whether observations of pulmonary dysfunction measured by epidemiologists have relevance to the clinical situation.

## *Epidemiological Observations*

Epidemiologists, in contrast to clinicians, study large numbers of individuals in so-called 'normal populations' over long periods of time. Understandably, the three relevant areas of disease studied by epidemiologists are cardiovascular disease, cancer, and what was called chronic bronchitis and has come to be described as COPD. Important studies include the classical Framingham Study in America [4] and more recently the Multiple Risk Factor Intervention Trial in America [5]. Two important and longstanding studies in this country are the Whitehall Study [6], in which a large group of male civil servants in London had been studied over a 20-year period, and the West of Scotland study of two populations, that of Renfrew and Paisley [7], which continues to yield interesting data. In order to describe these large numbers, the powerful tool of statistics is used. Data are nearly always derived from questionnaires, sometimes self-applied. In respiratory disease, the tried and tested MRC questionnaire on chronic bronchitis, first devised in the late 1950s and subsequently modified, is still in use [8]. In many studies, a simple and reproducible measurement such as an electrocardiogram, a blood test or a measure of respiratory function, such as $FEV_1$ or FVC (forced vital capacity) have been made.

The epidemiological studies of large cohorts of 'well populations' from which subsets have been generated have, in the main, concerned chronic air flow limitation (in COPD) on the one hand, and, of course, coronary heart disease on the other. I think it is because these two diseases were studied separately that until quite recently the two major groupings of epidemiologists have tended to pay scant regard the one to the other. Increasingly, their separate areas of interest have independently yielded the observation that there seems to be a relationship between measured or symptomatic respiratory impairment and coronary heart disease mortality.

At a meeting of the National Institutes of Health to consider mortality trends in COPD held at Bethesda, Maryland, in 1989, Prof. Frank Speizer [9], an eminent respiratory epidemiologist, commented on the importance of $FEV_1$ as an independent risk factor and predictor of mortality in cardiovascular disease. This observation came from groups studying COPD mortality. In summing up the data presented, he commented that such studies clearly showed that poor pulmonary function is an important predictor of mortality of all causes in both smokers and nonsmokers. This observation is not new, it had been suggested in two sets of the Framingham Study 8–9 years before the Bethesda meeting, but confirmation of this observation from a number of studies with excellent quality assurance for pulmonary function tests was regarded as important. Speizer commented that the relationship between poor lung function and premature mortality in COPD was not at all surprising in smokers, but was unanticipated in nonsmokers, and support for Speizer's overall observation came in detail from the Multiple Risk Factor Intervention Trial [5], which used the longitudinal analysis of all participants. Detailed analysis of specific intervention and 'usual control' groups showed decreased respiratory function to be an independent risk factor for coronary heart disease.

Kuller et al. [5] argue that the level of pulmonary function should be considered an established coronary heart disease risk factor. In so doing, however, they pointed out that impaired respiratory function may be highly correlated with other risk factors and may therefore confound the apparent association with coronary heart disease or total mortality.

Talkman and Comstock [10], from Johns Hopkins Hospital, studied respiratory factors on mortality in a 35,000 population in Washington County, Maryland. They noted the usual association between mortality and cigarette smoking, but also commented that a major observation of their study was that 'all cause', as well as cardiovascular disease and COPD mortality, is significantly more often found in subjects with ventilatory impairment independent of smoking status. They tried to explain reduction of pulmonary function as a consequence of cardiac failure. As $FEV_1$, $FEV_1/FVC$ percentage, and FVC had been measured, simple data which may distinguish lung from airway dysfunction were available. They argued that lung congestion would lead to decreased FVC and found that FVC and $FEV_1$ were decreased, but logistical regression showed that FVC percentage predicted fell out of the regression at the third step of the equation, leaving $FEV_1$ apparently a much more important risk factor. An alternative explanation to the relationship with coronary heart disease, therefore, seemed to be that of repeated inflammation, leading to airways obstructive disease which, added to the effect of lung ageing, makes for persistent arterial hypoxaemia which, they argued, constitutes a hazard for the emergence of coronary heart disease and thus mortality.

Another important epidemiological observation concerning airway disease was made at the Bethesda Meeting by Prof. Becklake of McGill University [11]. Using European data derived from longitudinal work studies in those exposed to dust and fumes in certain industrial processes over long periods of time, she suggested that industrial air pollution is a direct cause of COPD, controlling for age, sex and cigarette smoking. The analysis depended on careful spirometry on an annual basis, which was carried out on the work groups who were divided into smokers and nonsmokers and whose degree of exposure had been measured. Since confirmatory pathology was often available in this study, Prof. Becklake made an important contribution to the belief that industrial pollution per se can lead to inflammatory airway disease.

Respiratory impairment, as evidenced both by measurement and symptomatology, has been noted in further analysis of the Whitehall Study [12] and in a study by a collaborative group whose populations included the Whitehall Civil Service Study, the Paisley and Renfrew populations [13] and two American populations, selected on a work basis. The original MRC Chronic Bronchitis Questionnaire [8] had been usefully modified, such that a particular question regarding breathlessness when walking on the level was included. Pulmonary function was assessed by the percentage $FEV_1$ relative to predicted normal $FEV_1$.

Seventeen hundred and seventy-five deaths from coronary heart disease occurring over a 10-year period were analysed. The current smoking status of the four groups varied from 42 to 63%; phlegm production from 16 to 30% and dyspnoea when walking on the level from 6 to 14%. Statistical analysis showed that breathlessness when walking on the level was consistently and significantly associated with mortality in all studies.

One third of men reporting breathlessness were also found to have significantly reduced $FEV_1$. Of the group analysed, 50% had evidence of coronary heart disease at entry. Regression analysis left dyspnoea when walking on the level as the most statistically significant factor in predicting mortality, closely followed by $FEV_1$. The authors suggest that the presence of breathlessness should be attributed to coronary heart disease because of the emergence of dyspnoea as the most statistically significant factor. In her analysis of the Whitehall Civil Servant group, Dr. Ebi-Kryston [14] had suggested $FEV_1$ as the most important independent risk factor for coronary heart disease in males and had also found breathlessness when walking on the level equally predictive. She pointed out that neither observation was original but that evidence was accumulating to stress their validity.

In summary, from clinical observations and from epidemiological studies it seems that there is a good case for simple pulmonary function measurement in sharpening clinical focus in the prognosis of coronary heart disease.

## *References*


1 Collins JV, Clark TJH, Brown DJ: Airways function in healthy subjects and in patients with left heart disease. Clin Sci 1975;49:217–228.

2 Coates G, Powels ACP, Morrison SC, Sutton JR, Webber CE, Zylak CJ: The effects of intravenous infusion of saline on lung density, lung volumes, nitrogen washout, computed tomographic scans and chest radiographs in humans. Am Rev Respir Dis 1983;127:91–96.

3 Wilhelmsen L, Tibblin G, Grimby G, Bjure J, Ekstrom-Jodel B, Aurell M: Relationship between dyspnoea and later manifestations of clinical coronary heart disease and death; in Giuntini C, Panuccio P (eds): Cardiac Lung. Proceedings of an International Congress, Firenze 1976. Padova, Piccin Editore, 1979.

4 Kannel WB: Coronary risk factors. Recent highlights from the Framingham Study. Aust NZ J Med 1976;6:373–386.

5 Kuller LH, Ockene JK, Townsend M, Browner W, Meilahn E, Wentworth DM: The epidemiology of pulmonary function and COPD mortality in the Multiple Risk Factor Intervention Trial. Am Rev Respir Dis 1989;140:S76–S81.

6 Reid DD, Brett GZ, Hamilton PJS, Jarrett RJ, Keene H, Rose G: Cardiorespiratory disease and diabetes among middle-aged male civil servants. A study of screening and intervention. Lancet 1974;i:469–473.

7 Hawthorne VM, Gillies CR, McLean DS: Monitoring health in Scotland. Int J Epidemiol 1975;1:369–374.

8 Medical Research Council Questionnaire on Respiratory Symptoms and Instructions for its Use. London, Medical Research Council, 1966.

9 Speizer FE: Prognosis of chronic obstructive pulmonary disease. Am Rev Respir Dis 1989;140:S106–S107.

10 Talkman MS, Comstock WG: Respiratory risk factors in mortality: Longitudinal studies in Washington County, Maryland. Am Rev Respir Dis 1989;140:S56–S63.

11 Becklake MR: Occupational exposures: Evidence for a causal association with chronic obstructive pulmonary disease. Am Rev Respir Dis 1989;140:S85–S91.
12 Ebi-Kryston KL: Predicting 15-year chronic bronchitis mortality in the Whitehall Study. J Epidemiol Community Health 1989;43:168–172.
13 Hole DJ, Gillies CR, Chopra C, Hawthorne VM: Passive smoking in cardiorespiratory health in a general population in the West of Scotland. Br Med J 1989;299:423–427.
14 Ebi-Kryston KL: Respiratory symptoms in pulmonary function as predictors of ten-year mortality from respiratory disease, cardiovascular disease and all other causes in the Whitehall Study. J Clin Epidemiol 1988;41:251–260.

Dr. A.J.S. Gardiner, Monklands District General Hospital,
Airdrie, Lanarkshire ML6 0JS (UK)

Weetman DF, Wood D (eds): Risk Factors for Cardiovascular Disease in Non-Smokers. Int. Workshop, Washington, Tyne and Wear, 1991. Basel, Karger, 1993, pp 57–62

# Hypertension as a Risk Factor for Cardiovascular Disease

*R. Wilkinson*

Department of Nephrology, Freeman Hospital, Newcastle upon Tyne, UK

## *Blood Pressure Distribution in the Population*

Blood pressure in the whole population shows a Gaussian distribution with a tail at the upper end so that the definition of hypertension becomes difficult and to a certain extent empirical. As will be discussed, the risk of cardiovascular disease increases progressively from the low end of the normal distribution of blood pressure right through to higher levels. It is emphasized therefore that it is better to discuss blood pressure levels than to apply an artificial definition of hypertension; however, for practical clinical purposes, a definition is useful and that most commonly accepted is: 'the level of blood pressure at which treatment does more good than harm' [1].

## *Vascular Disease and Hypertension*

Hypertension leads to two major sets of changes in the vascular system. The smooth muscle in the walls of muscular resistance vessels hypertrophies in the face of an increased stress on the muscle from the higher blood pressure and this leads to a gradual narrowing of the lumen as the vessel wall thickens. This narrowing predisposes to tissue ischaemia, especially in the kidney. In addition, the hypertension traumatizes the intima of blood vessels, leading to platelet deposition on the traumatized area and subsequent atheromatous plaque formation, which predisposes to vascular occlusion both directly and by encouraging thrombus formation. As a result of these vascular changes, the clinical manifestations of vascular disease are increased in patients with hypertension. The commonest complication of hypertension is myocardial infarction, which occurs approximately twice as often as the next most common complication, stroke. Peripheral vascular disease is common in patients with hypertension, and heart failure and renal failure develop in severe cases.

### *The Quantitative Risk of Increased Blood Pressure*

Life insurance company statistics have shown that in patients aged 35 with only slightly increased blood pressure (to 130/95 mm Hg), life expectancy is reduced by 4 years from 76.5 to 72.5 years; when the blood pressure is 140/95 mm Hg, life expectancy is reduced to 67.5 years, and when the blood pressure is 150/100 mm Hg, the life expectancy is reduced to 60 years. These figures were of course obtained between the years 1925 and 1954 when there was no satisfactory treatment for mild hypertension and indeed even now such levels of blood pressure would not normally be treated. Subsequently, prospective data have been accumulated from the longitudinal survey of the population of Framingham, a small town in America, and this shows that for each 10-year age group 45–54, 55–64 and 65–74 there is an approximate doubling of the mortality rate in patients with hypertension compared to those without hypertension [2]. The absolute rate of mortality and morbidity is of course much lower in younger patients whatever the blood pressure but for any age there is a steady increase in morbidity and mortality with increasing levels of blood pressure.

A useful quantitation of the risk of hypertension in subjects between the ages of 35 and 64 years was provided by a population survey in South Wales which showed that at any level of blood pressure the risk in men was approximately double that in women. For men the risk of cardiovascular death or non-fatal stroke or myocardial infarction was 7.7/1,000 person years when the diastolic blood pressure was below 90 mm Hg, 19.3/1,000 person years when the diastolic pressure was between 90 and 109 mm Hg and 68.5/1,000 person years in patients with diastolic blood pressure of 110 mm Hg or more [3].

In industrialized societies there is a steady increase in systolic and diastolic blood pressures up to the age of approximately 60 years; beyond this, systolic pressure continues to rise but diastolic pressure plateaus and even falls with advancing age. This has been looked on as the normal pattern for blood pressure, but it has been shown in the Framingham survey in America [4] that the elderly with hypertension are at greater risk of cardiovascular death and morbidity than normotensive elderly subjects.

## *Factors Influencing Blood Pressure*

### *Heredity*

There is quite a strong inherited element in hypertension and work is in progress which is attempting to identify genetic markers for this predisposition to hypertension. It is thought that even with a genetic predisposition to hypertension, the hypertension may not develop unless environmental factors also predispose to the rise in blood pressure [5].

### *Obesity*

The Framingham survey has shown that blood pressure is high in obese subjects and several studies have shown that weight reduction is accompanied by a fall in blood pressure [6].

### *Alcohol*

In the late 1970s it was first noted that patients attending hypertension clinics had an increased incidence of abnormalities of liver function. This has since been confirmed in studies which demonstrated that patients who took more than 3 units of alcohol per day showed an increased incidence of hypertension. It has now been demonstrated that if alcohol intake is reduced then blood pressure falls [7].

### *Salt*

Comparisons of blood pressure in populations around the world with different intakes of salt have shown a correlation for populations between salt intake and blood pressure. Until recently it has been difficult to demonstrate such a correlation within populations, probably because the spread of salt intake was too small to allow significant relationships to be established. Recent studies have, however, confirmed a relationship between sodium intake and the rise in blood pressure with age within populations [8]. Furthermore, although there is some conflicting evidence, a review of published studies showed that a reduction in salt intake by 100 mol/day was accompanied by a reduction in diastolic blood pressure of about 10 mm Hg in hypertensive subjects [9].

### *Exercise*

Although blood pressure rises acutely during exercise, blood pressure falls in the period following the exercise and it has been shown that regular exercise is associated with lower blood pressure levels [10]. The management of hypertension should therefore include advice on obesity, alcohol intake, exercise habits and salt intake.

## *Evidence that Lowering Blood Pressure Can Reduce the Risk of Vascular Disease*

It was demonstrated in the mid-1950s that the treatment of malignant hypertension was beneficial and this was fairly easy to establish because without treatment 90% of patients were dead within a year. In the late 1960s it was established that the treatment of moderate hypertension reduced mortality: in a study in the Veterans' Administration Hospitals in the United States it was shown that morbidity from vascular disease could be halved with treatment [11]. However, two-thirds of deaths due to myocardial infarction occur at diastolic pressures below 110 mm Hg and one-half occur at diastolic pressures below 100 mm Hg. Similarly, three-quarters of strokes occur at diastolic blood pressures below 110 mm Hg and one-quarter at diastolic pressures below 100 mm Hg. Attention therefore has to be paid to the treatment of milder levels of blood pressure and it has proved more difficult to demonstrate benefit at these lower levels of pressure.

A large trial undertaken by the Medical Research Council (UK) in patients with mild hypertension (diastolic blood pressures between 90 and 110 mm Hg) showed that the number of strokes could be reduced to approximately one-half but there was unfortunately no evidence of benefit in preventing myocardial infarction [12]. This may well be because hypertension is responsible for only approximately 20% of the risk of myocardial infarction, with hyperlipidaemia accounting for approximately 20%, smoking for 20% and hereditary factors for about 35%. Hence, control of blood pressure alone could not be expected to reduce the risk of myocardial infarction dramatically.

Interestingly, it has been demonstrated that reduction of blood pressure in the elderly is accompanied by quite a marked reduction in the risk of myocardial infarction and stroke [13]. This supports the hypothesis that the rise in blood pressure seen in old age is not a physiological phenomenon.

## *How Well Is Blood Pressure Controlled in the Community?*

It has been estimated that only approximately 50% of patients with elevated blood pressure are known; of these only about one-half are on treatment and of those on treatment only about one-half are well controlled. Hypertension is usually asymptomatic and will only be detected by routine checking of blood pressure: studies have shown that the only effective way to achieve this is if the general practitioner or practice nurse checks the blood pressure of every patient who attends a surgery. It is only necessary to rescreen in patients with normal blood pressure after about 10 years. If the diastolic pressure is between 90 and 99 mm Hg, then the patient should probably be rescreened in 4 years and if it is mildly elevated at between 100 and 109 mm Hg, then the patient should be rescreened within 6 months, usually at a month and again at 3 months.

The benefits from the treatment of mild hypertension are small and it has been argued that the disadvantages of labelling a patient as hypertensive may outweigh these small benefits. Early reports suggested that the diagnosis of hypertension was followed by increased absenteeism, impaired marital adjustment and a lower sense of well-being. However, it has subsequently been shown that these disadvantages can be avoided by personal follow-up which gives the patient the feeling that the problem has been dealt with and is not a cause for worry.

## *References*


1 Pickering G: Hypertension: Definitions, natural histories and consequences; in Laragh JH, Brenner BM (eds.): Hypertension: Pathophysiology, Diagnosis and Management. New York, Raven Press, 1990, chapt 1, pp 3–16.

2 Wolf PA, Kannel WB, Cupples LA, D'Agostino RB: Risk factor interaction in cardiovascular and cerebrovascular disease; in Furlan AJ (ed): The Heart and Stroke: Exploring Mutual Cerebrovascular and Cardiovascular Issues. Berlin, Springer, 1987, pp 331–355.

3 Miall WE: Follow-up study of arterial pressure in the population of a Welsh mining valley. BMJ 1959;ii:1204–1207.

4 Kannel WB: Evaluation of cardiovascular risk in the elderly: The Framingham study. Bull NY Acad Med 1978;54:573–591.

5 Miall WE, Oldham PD: The hereditary factor in arterial blood pressure. BMJ 1963; i:75–78.

6 Kannel WB, Sorlie P: Hypertension in Framingham; in Paul O (ed): Epidemiology and Control of Hypertension. Miami, Symposia Specialists, 1975, pp 553–592.

7 Potter JF, Beevers DG: Pressor effect of alcohol in hypertension. Lancet 1984;i:119–122.

8 Intersalt Cooperative Research Group: Intersalt: An international study of electrolyte excretion and blood pressure. Results for 24-hour urinary sodium and potassium excretion. BMJ 1988;297:319–328.

9 Morgan T, Nowson C: The role of sodium restriction in the management of hypertension. Can J Physiol Pharmacol 1986;64:786–792.

10 Paffenbarger RS, Wing AL, Hyde RT, Jung DL: Physical activity and incidence of hypertension in college alumni. Am J Epidemiol 1983;117:245–257.

11 Veterans' Administration Cooperative Study Group on Antihypertensive agents: Effects of treatment on morbidity in hypertension. II. Results in patients with diastolic blood pressure averaging 90 through 114 mm Hg. JAMA 1970;213:1143–1152.

12 Medical Research Council Working Party: MRC trial of treatment of mild hypertension: Principal results. BMJ 1985;291:97–104.

13 Dahlof B, Lindholm LH, Hansson L, Schersten B, Ekbom T, Webster PO: Morbidity and mortality in the Swedish Trial in Old Patients with Hypertension (STOP-Hypertension). Lancet 1991;338:1281–1284.

Prof. R. Wilkinson, Department of Nephrology, Freeman Hospital,
Newcastle upon Tyne NE7 7DN (UK)

## *Discussion*

*Weetman* (Sunderland): In the Framingham study, was it not concluded that the increased risk associated with obesity was attributable to impaired glucose tolerance in type 2 diabetes?

*Wilkinson* (Newcastle upon Tyne): Although it is difficult to separate out individual risk factors, it has been shown clearly that obesity itself is an independent factor in raised blood pressure: it has been universally demonstrated that reducing weight lowers blood pressure.

Weetman DF, Wood D (eds): Risk Factors for Cardiovascular Disease in Non-Smokers. Int. Workshop, Washington, Tyne and Wear, 1991. Basel, Karger, 1993, pp 63–71

# Diabetes and 'Syndrome X'

*K.G.M.M. Alberti*

Department of Medicine, University of Newcastle upon Tyne, UK

Most people would consider that diabetes is a raised blood glucose concentration, but of course there is much more to it than this. There are two main types of diabetes; first the insulin-dependent type (insulin-dependent diabetes mellitus: IDDM), which was formerly known as 'juvenile-onset' diabetes [1]. The second major type of diabetes is non-insulin-dependent diabetes mellitus (NIDDM), which used to be known as 'maturity-onset' diabetes, as it occurs mainly in older people. This latter disease is much commoner than the insulin-dependent type: around the world as a whole, about 85–95% of diabetic patients have NIDDM.

IDDM is very much a disease of the north – the further north you go, the more of it there is: if you happen to be a Lapp, you have something like a 3-fold greater risk of developing IDDM than if you came from the north-east of England, and the rate here is 5 times greater than that in the south of France, and 10 times greater risk than if you were from China, so there are some considerable geographical variations in the incidence of IDDM. Recent data from Northern England show an annual incidence of 14/100,000 for IDDM [2], with a national prevalence of about 0.25%.

In England, a maximal estimate is that about 2% of the population have NIDDM, of whom half are undiagnosed. In one sense it is rather like hypertension: you do not get symptoms until late on in the disease. Thus many people are walking around with their condition undiagnosed. This is in distinct contrast to IDDM, which is characterized by a lesion in the B cells of the islets of Langerhans in the pancreas. The insulin deficiency arises because the B cell can no longer make insulin, so the hormone has to be replaced therapeutically, hence the term insulin-dependent. The NIDDM patients differ in that they have insulin, but their main metabolic feature is that it does not work properly, so-called insulin resistance. The insulin levels in such a NIDDM patient are usually higher than those in normal subjects, but they still cannot control the blood glucose properly, so there would be a raised blood glucose. Insulin resistance is thus one of the main features of NIDDM. The people most at risk from cardiovascular diseases, i.e. those aged 40 years and older, also include virtually all those affected by NIDDM.

If diabetes was just raised blood glucose, it could be treated very easily, but there are more features of the disease than this. Lundbaek, who was a distinguished Professor of Medicine in Denmark, used to give the following definition of diabetes: 'A spot in the eye in twenty years' time.' In other words, he was referring to the fact that once you have diabetes you are at risk of developing the long-term complications. These include kidney damage (nephropathy), nerve damage (neuropathy), eye damage (retinopathy) and long-term large blood vessel disease (macroangiopathy) with peripheral gangrene, particularly of the feet.

The current view about complications is that the small blood vessels are affected. There is also microangiopathy affecting the eye. Diabetes is a leading cause of blindness. The kidney is also affected; diabetes in younger people is a leading cause of renal failure. Some patients exhibit neuropathy, which too may be related to small blood vessels, or could follow a direct attack on the nerve. Disease of the large blood vessels can also occur, leading to heart disease, cerebrovascular disease and peripheral vascular disease, all of which are of direct relevance to the main topic of this workshop. The extent of these secondary effects on blood vessels is extremely important because they represent the leading cause of death in diabetic people. In all diabetic patients, ischaemic heart disease is by far the major cause of death; cerebrovascular disease also contributes appreciably [3]. Renal failure is most frequently encountered in the IDDM patients (table 1).

Macrovascular disease is the major problem for diabetic patients. The whole population has to die from some cause, and for most it is macrovascular disease. If you have diabetes you die sooner from macrovascular disease. Table 2 considers the prevalence rates that were identified in the Framingham study [5]. There are three main sorts of macrovascular disease: cerebrovascular disease causing stroke and transient ischaemic attacks (TIAs); intermittent claudication, which is peripheral vascular disease; and then coronary vascular disease. For men, it is the number of events (i.e. not deaths) that is greatly increased in diabetes compared with non-diabetic people, and again it is mainly NIDDM patients who are affected. Non-diabetic women have lower rates than men, particularly for intermittent claudication and coronary events, but this advantage is lost in those who have diabetes. In effect, diabetic women assume the male level of risk for macrovascular disease, so that they suffer an enormously increased relative risk for cardiac disease, cerebrovascular disease, etc.

*Table 1.* Causes of death in diabetes mellitus

| | IDDM, % | NIDDM, %[1] | NIDDM, %[2] |
|---|---|---|---|
| Cardiovascular disease | 15 | 58 | 37 |
| Cerebrovascular disease | 3 | 12 | 22 |
| Renal disease | 55 | 3 | 3 |
| Diabetic 'coma' | 4 | 3 | 3 |
| Infections | 10 | 4 | 8 |
| Malignancy | 0 | 11 | 10 |

[1] And IDDM figures from Marks and Krall [3].
[2] From Panzram [4].

*Table 2.* Average annual incidence (age-adjusted) per 1,000 specified cardiovascular events over a 20-year period in diabetic and non-diabetic individuals [adapted from 5]

| | Males | | Females | |
|---|---|---|---|---|
| | diabetic | non-diabetic | diabetic | non-diabetic |
| Cardiovascular disease | 39 | 19 | 27 | 10 |
| CVD deaths | 17 | 9 | 17 | 4 |
| Congestive heart failure | 8 | 4 | 11 | 2 |
| Ischaemic heart disease | 25 | 15 | 18 | 7 |
| Intermittent claudication | 13 | 3 | 8 | 1 |
| Cerebrovascular disease | 5 | 2 | 6 | 2 |

The risk factors for heart disease in the general population can be categorized into those we cannot avoid, such as age, sex and family history, and modifiable ones, such as cigarette smoking, hypertension, hyperlipidaemia, a sedentary lifestyle, obesity and diabetes. In diabetes, many other risk factors are present. Table 3 presents findings, from Germany, summarizing the risk factors for macrovascular disease in patients with NIDDM and in the general population [6]. The definition of hyperlipidaemia was very strict, so perhaps the figures should be a lot higher to reflect the true risk: twice as many NIDDM patients had hyperlipidaemia as in the general population; the very high cholesterol levels, over 300 mg/dl or 7.8 mmol/l, were the same in both groups; triglycerides were higher; uric acid (which appears to be a risk factor, although the mechanism is obscure) was also higher. There was a 53% incidence of hypertension in the diabetic group (we found much the same figure from our studies in Newcastle), which

*Table 3.* Cardiovascular risk factors at diagnosis in NIDDM in Germany (D15 study) [data from 6]

| Risk factor | NIDDM, % | General population, % |
|---|---|---|
| Hyperlipidaemia | 17.6 | 7.6 |
| Cholesterol > 7.8 mmol/l | 3.5 | 3.7 |
| Triglycerides elevated | 11.3 | 3.4 |
| Hyperuricaemia | 22.5 | 3.8 |
| Hypertension | 53.0 | 17.3 |
| Smoking | 34.0 | 30.3 |

relates to 17% in the non-diabetic German population. The diabetic subjects smoked as much as the general population.

Thus diabetic people have higher than normal rates for hypertension and hyperlipidaemia, which are the key risk factors. It has become apparent recently that various risk factors appear to cluster in diabetes. Very often people with diabetes (or just individuals with an abnormal glucose tolerance) have hypertension, dyslipidaemia (particularly high triglycerides and a low HDL cholesterol), and central obesity. Central obesity is typified by people with big abdomens: they are the high-risk people. It is possible to identify central obesity from measurements of the waist/hip ratio, which we do routinely now in our subjects. Central obesity is the male form of obesity, where a large amount of fat accumulates in and around the abdomen, so that the adipose tissue within the abdominal cavity drains directly to the liver through the portal venous system. This could be the trigger for the increased cardiovascular risk. In contrast, the female type of obesity, gynaecoid obesity, is characterized by a large backside and hips, with less fat around the waist: these patients are not at increased cardiovascular risk. Total body fat is not important, it is the distribution of the fat.

When the characteristics described above cluster together, they are all associated with insulin resistance and high insulin levels in the blood. The term 'Syndrome X' has been used to describe this clustering [7]. It is not yet known whether or not the clustering arises by chance; alternatively, it could be causally related to the increased cardiovascular risk.

If you eliminate all the known risk factors, you still have a 2-fold excess in risk, so there is something about diabetes itself that increases the risk for macrovascular disease. Why is this? The range of possible mechanisms will be considered next.

(1) With respect to the possible cellular mechanisms of dyslipoproteinaemia, there are two or three things which could be relevant. In diabetes there is often a combination of a high LDL cholesterol, a high

*Table 4.* Effect of 1 year of treatment in new NIDDM subjects [data from 9]

| | Initial | One year |
|---|---|---|
| BMI, $kg/m^2$ | $28.3 \pm 0.5$ | $27.5 \pm 0.6$* |
| HbA1, % | $10.7 \pm 0.3$ | $8.2 \pm 0.2$* |
| Blood pressure, mm Hg | | |
| Systolic | $153 \pm 3$ | $151 \pm 2$ |
| Diastolic | $86 \pm 1$ | $83 \pm 1$ |
| Total cholesterol, m*M* | $6.2 \pm 0.2$ | $6.0 \pm 0.1$ |
| HDL cholesterol, m*M* | $1.0 \pm 0.1$ | $1.0 \pm 0.1$ |
| Triglycerides, m*M* | $3.1 \pm 0.3$ | $2.7 \pm 0.2$ |

* $p < 0.05$.

triglyceride and a low HDL cholesterol, and it is the combination, particularly of the last two, that seems to be a very powerful predictor [8]. Furthermore, the lipoprotein particles are abnormal in composition, with a lot of IDL (intermediate density lipoproteins), which may be interacting abnormally with macrophages, and also with the arterial wall.

If one considers the lipid risk factors and the high prevalence of dyslipoproteinaemia in 130 new diabetics in Newcastle (table 4); values were recorded when they were first seen and then 1 year later. The index of diabetes control is represented by HbA (i.e. glycated haemoglobin), which improved greatly over the year. However, it was the only thing that did improve, because readings for total cholesterol (mean value 6 mmol/l, which is really quite high), HDL cholesterol, triglycerides and systolic blood pressure all failed to improve. Thus a considerable risk persisted in our diabetic patients because the lipids and blood pressure were abnormal. With respect to obesity, the BMI was slightly lower, but they had lost on average only about 250 g in 1 year.

(2) With respect to haemostatic changes, there are many abnormalities (table 5). These involve platelets, in terms of aggregation, thromboxane release, and growth factor release; there are clotting factor abnormalities, including raised fibrinogen levels and the concentrations of factor VII and factor VIII are abnormal, fibrinolysis decreases, and the red cells are more rigid. Thus there are many reasons for these factors to be involved in this increased risk of macrovascular disease in diabetes.

(3) Most NIDDM patients exhibit hyperinsulinaemia and high insulin levels have been suggested to be causative for atheroma [10]. One possibility is that insulin exerts a direct growth factor effect on cell walls. There have been some large epidemiological studies that have concluded that there is an association between raised insulin and excess macrovascular

*Table 5.* Atheroma-promoting haemostatic changes in NIDDM

| | |
|---|---|
| 1. | Platelet dysfunction<br>Increased aggregation<br>Thromboxane production<br>Growth factor release |
| 2. | Clotting factor abnormalities<br>Raised fibrinogen<br>Increased factor VII and VIII activities<br>Decreased fibrinolysis |
| 3. | Cell-like forces<br>Red blood corpuscle rigidity |

disease, but these are not entirely convincing for a number of reasons, including the weakness of the associations. If one attempts to find direct evidence, for example by taking biopsy samples from the arteries of hyperinsulinaemic diabetics or animal models, more triglyceride is found in the arteries as well as muscle [11]. Although it is possible to generate atheroma in these animals with hyperinsulinaemia, one has to be careful in the interpretation of these findings.

(4) It is possible that protein glycation may be involved with the macrovascular disease in diabetes [12]. As was made clear from Dr. Bruckdorfer's paper, in the presence of high concentrations of glucose in the circulation, there will be the formation of covalent bonds to protein (in fact to any free amino groups) by a non-enzymatic reaction. Low density lipoproteins will be glycated, which will then bind abnormally to receptors and are picked up preferentially by macrophages. This could be the mechanism. Furthermore, if lysine binds glucose actually in the aorta, via epsilon amino groups, there will be a very abnormal advanced glycosylation end-product macrophage interaction, and you set a sequence of events in process where myosin itself gets glycated. Cell membranes may also be glycated, resulting in much damage through glycation. This sequence is speculative, and not yet supported by direct evidence, but if it were to occur, the last step would be where insulin, acting as a growth factor, could compound the vascular lesion.

(5) It has been suggested that in diabetes there is more endothelial cell injury, partly due to hypertension, partly due to sorbitol which is formed from glucose when there is an excess of glucose [13]. The resulting endothelial cell injury, perhaps by an osmotic mechanism, and perhaps partly through hypoxia, results in foam cell activation, and insulin may well be directly involved in this step, glycated lipoproteins too may be involved, so that the final step is a pronounced smooth muscle cell

proliferation. Again in this final step, insulin may be a major growth factor with other growth factors being involved as well.

In conclusion, there is a large increase in macrovascular disease in diabetes; unfortunately, it is not just a simple enhancement of normal risk factors. These are involved, of course, but there is also the additional diabetes-specific risk, whose possible mechanism has been discussed above. One cannot escape the impression that with respect to the mechanism of the vascular problems of diabetics, we are really scratching away at the tip of a very big iceberg, but it is a very important one, because it is the main cause of death in diabetes.

## *References*

1 WHO Expert Committee on Diabetes mellitus: Second Report. Tech Rep Ser No 646. Geneva, WHO, 1980.

2 Crow YJ, Alberti KGMM, Parkin JM: Insulin-dependent diabetes in childhood and material deprivation in Northern England, 1977–1986. BMJ 1991;303:158–160.

3 Marks HH, Krall LP: Onset, course and prognosis and mortality in diabetes mellitus; in Marble A, White P, Bradley RF, Krall LP (eds): Joslin's Diabetes mellitus, ed, 11. Philadelphia, Lea & Febiger, 1981, pp 209–254.

4 Panzram G: Mortality and survival in type 2 (non-insulin-dependent) diabetes mellitus. Diabetologia 1987;30:123–131.

5 Kannel WB, McGee DL: Diabetes and cardiovascular disease. The Framingham study. JAMA 1979;241:2035–2038.

6 Hanefeld M, Fischer S, Schmechel H, Rothe G, Schulze J, Dude H, Schwanebeck U, Julius U: Diabetes intervention study. Multi-intervention trial in newly diagnosed NIDDM. Diabetes Care 1991;14:308–317.

7 Reaven GM: Role of insulin resistance in human disease. Diabetes 1988;37:1595–1607.

8 Castelli WP: The triglyceride issue: A view from Framingham. Am Heart J 1986;112:432–437.

9 Marsiaj HI, Catalano C, Sum CF, Home PD, Alberti KGMM: Management of newly diagnosed non-insulin-dependent (type 2) diabetes mellitus: A retrospective audit. Diab Res Clin Pract 1991;12:129–136.

10 Stout RW: The role of insulin in atherosclerosis in diabetics and non-diabetics. Diabetes 1983;30 (suppl 2):54–57.

11 Falholt K, Alberti KGMM, Heding LG: Aorta and muscle metabolism in pigs with peripheral hyperinsulinaemia. Diabetologia 1985;28:32–37.

12 Vlassara H: Non-enzymatic glycosylation; in Alberti KGMM, Krall LP (eds): Diabetes Annual 6. Amsterdam, Elsevier, 1991, pp 371–389.

13 Hotta N, Sakamoto N: Aldose reductase inhibitors; in Alberti KGMM, Krall LP (eds): Diabetes Annual 5. Amsterdam, Elsevier, 1990, pp 330–361.

14 Dean JD, Jones CDH, Hutchison SJ, Peters JR, Henderson AH: Hyperinsulinaemia and microvascular angina. Lancet 1991;337:456–457.

15 Jarrett RJ, Viberti GC, Argyropoulos A et al.: Microalbuminuria predicts mortality in non-insulin-dependent diabetes. Diabetic Med 1984;1:17–19.

Prof. K.G.M.M. Alberti, Department of Medicine, The Medical School, University of Newcastle upon Tyne, Newcastle upon Tyne NE2 4HH (UK)

## *Discussion*

*Bruckdorfer* (London): I was wondering whether you think the sorbitol pathway really has much importance. I understand the inhibitors, i.e. drugs that inhibit the pathway, have not been particularly effective either in the neuropathies or in any other aspects.

*Alberti* (Newcastle upon Tyne): No, I do not think they are a major factor, but I think they are one of several factors. I do not think we have given the drugs a fair trial. They have been given so far to people who already had early complications, used for 3 years, and then the conclusion has been reached that they do not work. Perhaps one should not expect them to work. Ideally, you need to give them to people at the beginning of diabetes and see if they will inhibit the development of complications. We have this enormous problem with macrovascular disease in NIDDM because the soonest we see a patient is 5 years after the onset of the disease, because of the lack of a reliable method for early diagnosis. Possibly the best solution would be to set up combined screening units for hypertension and NIDDM; cases could then be identified early and be followed before there are too many complications. In fact we are doing that now, and I think then we may start to see ways of preventing the macrovascular complications as well.

*Lorimer* (Glasgow): In cardiological terms, quite often you would use the term 'Syndrome X' to describe patients who have normal coronary arteries, and perhaps, or perhaps not, microvascular signs by some fault at the cellular level. Do you think that this particular group of people are relevant in diabetes?

*Alberti:* Yes. There has been interesting correspondence in *The Lancet* recently [14], because of the problems of the cardiologists using the wrong name for their syndrome! The diabetic term is also known as Reaven's syndrome after Gerry Reaven [7] in Stanford; he was not the first person to describe it, but he caught people at the right moment when he did. I think microvascular disease of the heart is important and Lundbaek, whom I mentioned with respect to the 'Spot in the eye in twenty years' time' described diabetic cardiomyopathy as 'small vessel disease of the heart with relatively normal coronaries', and even in 15-year-olds you can pick up ventricular dysfunction, so I think that lies behind it as well.

*Lorimer:* There have been some reports, have there not, of what the cardiologists would call 'syndrome X', in which there are abnormalities of insulin?

*Alberti:* Yes, that is what the Welshmen recently showed [12]: insulin insensitivity in their patients. However, you will find it in most diseases, if you look hard enough. When you get a sick person, they are generally secreting counter-regulatory hormones, and there is always some insulin resistance, so it is a little difficult to sort out.

*Salter* (Nottingham): Do you believe that the risk factors in IDDM are the same risk factors which are increasing the prevalence in NIDDM?

*Alberti:* I think largely I do. If IDDM patients can be kept alive long enough through their renal problems, we see the same outcomes. There are more and more deaths from CVD in IDDM patients in their 30s and 40s. There is a link-up with proteinuria, because proteinuria in diabetic people is predictive of death from cardiovascular disease [15], although the precise mechanism of the association is unclear; but it is found in both IDDM and in NIDDM. However, there is less dyslipidaemia in IDDM patients, but the other risk factors are probably the same, and they tend to be hyperinsulinaemic as well because of the way insulin is administered.

*Bruckdorfer:* On the question of insulin and its effects on the artery wall as far as lipid synthesis is concerned, you suggested, I think, that it was actually triglyceride synthesis which increased: now that would not be what you see in atherosclerosis, where there is accumulation of cholesterol. I was wondering where this triglyceride actually is: Is it perhaps associated with the abdomen tissue or media rather than the internal areas?

*Alberti:* It seems to be scattered all over the place, in fact, and we are still trying to sort out whether it is synthesized there or transported there. My colleagues in Denmark measured triglyceride rather than cholesterol because of the ease of measurement in arterial wall samples. What we are trying to do now is to see exactly where the fat is by histology, whether in the pigs or people they have studied there is a typical type of atheroma or if it is something quite different.

Weetman DF, Wood D (eds): Risk Factors for Cardiovascular Disease in Non-Smokers. Int. Workshop, Washington, Tyne and Wear, 1991. Basel, Karger, 1993, pp 72–85

# Design and Analysis of Epidemiological Studies

*Peter N. Lee*

Consultant in Epidemiology and Statistics, Sutton, Surrey, UK

This paper is concerned with the design and analysis of epidemiological studies. I will consider general issues that apply to all types of epidemiological study, although occasionally I will use illustrative examples drawn from an area of particular interest to me, the interpretation of the evidence on environmental tobacco smoke (ETS) and cardiovascular disease.

Firstly, I shall describe the five main types of epidemiological study, summarizing the main strengths and weaknesses of each type. I shall then expand on some of the problems of design and analysis of epidemiological studies.

## *Randomized Trials*

In a randomized study a group of healthy subjects is identified and then randomly divided into two groups, one of which is exposed to the agent of interest. The two groups are then followed up for some years to determine the proportions dying or becoming ill from the disease of interest. Unlike the other four types of study, which are observational in nature, randomized trials are experimental, i.e. whether or not a subject is exposed is under the control of the experimenter rather than being determined by the subject. Since the randomization process ensures that the two groups differ systematically only in respect of the exposure of interest, such studies have the enormous advantage of virtually eliminating the possibility, ever present in observational studies, that observed differences in risk between the groups being compared might be a result of differences in risk factors other than the exposure of interest. Randomized trials are, however, completely impractical for many types of exposure. For example, one cannot realistically persuade a group of nonsmokers to take part in a randomized trial of ETS exposure in which about half of them will be forced to spend some hours per day over a number of years in a smoky room.

Because randomized trials are not practicable for many of the types of risk factor discussed in this workshop, and because observational studies have many more problems in design, analysis and interpretation, I will concentrate in the rest of this paper on observational studies.

### *Prospective Studies*

In a prospective study, often referred to as a cohort study, a sample of the healthy living population is interviewed to determine the exposure of interest and other relevant risk factors and is then followed up for a period to see which subjects die or become ill from the disease of interest. In this type of study, subjects may be re-interviewed at intervals to obtain updated information on risk factors.

### *Case-Control Studies*

In a case-control study, often known as a retrospective study, information on the exposure of interest and on other relevant risk factors is obtained for 'cases' who have died from or are suffering from particular diseases and compared with those obtained for 'control' groups not suffering from these diseases. Control groups can either be a sample of the living population or can be people who have died or are suffering from certain diseases assumed to be unrelated to the risk factor under investigation (and who therefore should be representative of the living population in this respect).

Whereas in a prospective study it is straightforward to measure relative risk by comparing the risk of disease in the exposed group with that in the unexposed group, it is not straightforward to see how to do so in a case-control study where one is comparing frequency of exposure in those with the disease of interest and in those who do not have it. To see how this is done, consider a population consisting of $n_1$ unexposed individuals and $n_2$ exposed individuals of a given age, and suppose that in a short period of time there are $d_1$ deaths in the unexposed individuals and $d_2$

deaths in the exposed individuals. In the prospective study situation, the relative risk R is estimated by:

$$R = \frac{d_2/n_2}{d_1/n_1}, \quad \text{rearranging:} \quad R = \frac{d_2/d_1}{n_2/n_1}.$$

In a case-control study, $d_2/d_1$ can be estimated from the relative frequency of exposed and unexposed in the 'cases' and $n_2/n_1$ from the relative frequency of exposed and unexposed in the 'controls'. Strictly, the latter relative frequency is actually based on survivors from $n_1$ and $n_2$, but provided that deaths are only a small fraction of the population, the difference is trivial. Note, however, that although relative risk can be calculated in both types of study, absolute risk can only be calculated in prospective studies.

Both prospective and case-control studies have the disadvantage of being unrandomized, with the possibility of bias due to confounding by measured or unmeasured risk factors. Compared to prospective studies, case-control studies have a number of further disadvantages. First, there may be doubts as to whether the selected control group actually has exposure typical of the population at large. Second, if one measures current exposure, an association might be seen because presence of disease might affect exposure (e.g. people may change their diet when ill) rather than because exposure causes the disease, whereas if one records past exposure one is reliant on memory of the patient, or next of kin, which may be inaccurate. A third disadvantage of case-control studies involving patients rather than decedents is that surviving cases may be unrepresentative of all cases. Suppose, for example, that exposure has no effect on onset of disease, but actually reduces the probability of death for those with the disease. Here a case-control study would falsely conclude that exposure is harmful. A fourth disadvantage is that case-control studies produce results for only one disease whereas prospective studies automatically provide data for all causes of death.

There are, however, a number of practical disadvantages with prospective studies. One is the fact that case-control studies can produce results much faster than prospective studies, often in months compared with the 20+ years for some prospective studies, such as the British Doctors' Study [1] or the Framingham Study [2]. Another relates to the much larger number of subjects who need to be interviewed, and therefore the cost. Whereas in a case-control study one might typically interview 100, 200 or 300 controls to balance 100 cases, in a prospective study one may have had to interview 10,000 or even 100,000 subjects to end up with 100 who contract the disease of interest. Prospective studies are completely impractical for very rare diseases, although this is not a limitation for cardiovascular disease. Prospective studies may also be difficult to organize in countries where routine facilities are not available to determine whether specified individuals have died and, if so, from what cause: a problem in the USA or Germany, but not in the UK or Scandinavia. Prospective studies are also often much less convenient to organize than case-control studies, which can sometimes be conducted in a single hospital over a short period of time.

### *Cross-Sectional Studies*

These involve interviewing a representative sample and simultaneously determining presence of the disease of interest, the exposure of interest and other risk factors. Such studies are really only appropriate for study of reasonably common nonfatal conditions, e.g. cardiovascular symptoms such as angina. They have many of the problems of other types of observational studies, including the difficulty of distinguishing 'exposure causes disease' from 'exposure affected by disease'.

### *Ecological Correlation Studies*

Whereas the previous four types of study relate exposure and incidence of disease at the individual level, ecological correlation studies relate them at the group level. Thus one might correlate risk and exposure in different races, regions and countries (for example, breast cancer rate and total dietary fat intake were very highly correlated when data for 39 countries were plotted [3]) or one might correlate risk and exposure in the same population at different time points. While ecological correlation studies are considered of value in suggesting hypotheses and may also help to confirm or refute hypotheses, they are not generally considered to be primary evidence of a cause-and-effect relationship. There are a number of reasons why they do not provide the strength of evidence of prospective or case-control studies. For instance, if a correlation is found, one does not know whether those who died of the disease of interest were actually exposed to the agent of interest. Another reason is that information on all relevant confounding variables may not be available. Time correlations in particular are notorious for producing spurious associations, and are of especially dubious value for chronic diseases. It is quite possible that a factor may actually cause a disease but one may still observe disease incidence to be rising in a population at a time when exposure is falling, simply because risk is dependent primarily on past exposure. If one is not careful one ends up correlating incidence of a disease occurring predominantly in grandparents with exposure occurring predominantly in their grandchildren!

*Problems of Design and Analysis of Epidemiological Studies*

Rather than consider the problems of design and analysis of prospective and case-control studies separately, I will consider both issues simultaneously by looking at the various problems of inference that can arise and how they affect design and analysis of such studies. One general point to make is that analysis of these studies is not merely a matter of presenting estimates of risk in relation to exposure adjusted for relevant confounding factors, but also of considering each of the problems of inference that can arise formally and discussing their importance. Certainly it is not possible to conclude that an observed association indicates a cause-and-effect relationship unless all alternative possible explanations for it can be excluded. In practice, this may be difficult or impossible for evidence from many epidemiological studies.

*Chance*

Clearly one has to exclude the reasonable possibility that the observed association might be due to chance. From the point of view of design of a study, one must have enough deaths or cases to ensure that there is an adequate probability of picking up a difference in risk if one exists. Formal power calculations should be undertaken. In the context of ETS and heart disease it should be noted that only two of the published studies had a power greater than 10% to detect a relative risk of 1.2 [4]. Partly this was because many, if not all, of the studies were not specifically designed with this association in mind. When designing a study it should also be noted that larger numbers of subjects will be required if one wants to study the possibility that exposure might have differing effects in different subsets of the population.

When analyzing a study it is advisable to present not only probability (p) values but also confidence limits, so as to give a better indication of the variability of the relative risk estimate. When interpreting p values, it should be remembered that they are merely aids to judgement: some experimenters seem to base their conclusions simply on whether or not $p < 0.05$. This is very bad practice. In the first place, a low p value (e.g. $p = 0.001$) is much more convincing evidence of an association than is a less low p value (e.g. $p = 0.04$) so that the magnitude of the p value should be presented. Secondly, of course, even if chance can essentially be ruled out by a very low p value, the association might still be an artefact due to one or more of the various sources of bias discussed below.

A very important point to understand is that p values are only really appropriate if they relate to tests of hypotheses decided in advance. If detailed analysis from a large database shows a high risk of disease in left-handed blacks of low social class with a surviving grandmother, the associated p value, even if quite low, may simply reflect the fact that if enough analyses are performed, an association will almost certainly be found. Unless the p value is exceptionally low, taking into account the number of tests carried out, the association can at best be treated as a suggestion to be confirmed by further studies. Published papers frequently ignore this problem of 'data dredging' and place totally unfounded faith in the reality of such associations, just because they are statistically significant.

*Sequence of Events*

A false conclusion regarding effects of exposure can occur if in fact disease affects exposure. Thus, for example, an association has been observed between low cholesterol and some types of cancer simply because the presence of cancer reduced cholesterol levels. There is an obvious need in case-control studies to record past exposures. This may also apply, for some exposures, to prospective studies. Although prospective studies are usually conducted on overtly healthy individuals, some may have incipient undiagnosed disease that may affect some exposures. Where this seems a possibility it can be useful, during analysis, to study the association subdivided by time from the start of the study. Such a bias would reasonably be suspected if the association were strongly evident in the first year or two of the study, but not subsequently.

*Misclassification of Disease and Exposure*

This is a problem in all studies, though the magnitude of it will vary with the nature of the disease and the type of exposure considered. It is a well-known statistical fact that *random* misclassification of one or both of two variables being associated tends to result in the observed association being weaker than the true association. Random misclassification cannot explain an observed association. For an association to have arisen as an artefact of misclassification, a mechanism for *differential* misclassification has to exist. One possibility applicable to both prospective and case-control studies is that a disease caused by exposure may be misclassified as the disease of interest; for example, cancer at one site may metastasize to other sites, with some of these secondaries being falsely diagnosed as primaries. Another source of differential misclassification arises if knowledge of exposure may affect diagnosis. It has been documented, for example, that a part of the observed association between smoking and lung cancer arises because a smoker with lung cancer is more likely to be diagnosed as having lung cancer than is a nonsmoker with lung cancer [5]. Yet another source, applicable only to case-control studies, arises if knowledge of disease affects recall of exposure. Case-control studies looking at family history of disease as a possible risk factor are particularly vulnerable to this source of bias.

There are a number of implications of this for both design and analysis: data should be collected using the most accurate methods possible, the 'double-blind' technique should be used if feasible (i.e. the person diagnosing the disease should not know the exposure of interest, and the person reporting exposure should not be aware of the disease), and information should be sought on accuracy of the data collected (e.g. by using multiple measurements or multiple sources). In analysis, one should try to correct relative risk estimates for estimated misclassification or at least try to assess the likely relevance of misclassification.

*Inadequate Control Group*

The observation that cases with disease X have higher exposure than controls with disease Y is not only consistent with exposure increasing risk of X but also with it decreasing risk of Y. Unless the exposure of the controls is representative of the population at large, one cannot make reliable inferences as to whether exposure affects disease X. Although the above argument suggests that random population controls are ideal, hospital controls may have advantages for some studies. This is because reported exposure may well depend on where, when and by whom the information is given and use of suitable hospital controls tends to facilitate cases and controls being similar in these respects. The same principle of comparing like with like means that if data on cases are collected from next of kin, so also should be data on controls. In some studies, it may be of value to have more than one control group. Demonstration that exposure is high in cases, but similarly low in a number of control groups adds to the evidence that the association is not an artefact of a poor choice of controls.

*Nonresponse*

Only some subjects approached provide usable data, and the relative risk estimate may be biassed as a result. Suppose, for example, that in a case-control study, cases are personally interviewed in hospital and all or virtually all respond, while controls are interviewed by telephone or by mailed questionnaire and only a proportion respond. If exposed people tend to be less likely to respond, a spuriously positive relative risk will emerge. Data on proportion of nonresponse should be presented and the extent of possible bias considered.

In prospective studies, it is important to ensure that follow-up for deaths is as complete as possible if bias is to be avoided. Doll and Peto [1] in the British Doctor's study took enormous pains to try to follow all their sample (and lost less than 0.5%) because of worries about bias due to incomplete follow-up. In contrast, the two main prospective studies providing evidence on ETS and heart disease [6, 7] made no attempt to pursue subjects who left the original area where interviewing was conducted.

*Confounding*

Smokers have higher liver cirrhosis rates than nonsmokers, not because of any direct effect of smoking, but because smokers drink more than nonsmokers, and because alcohol predisposes to liver cirrhosis. Here, alcohol is said to confound the smoking/cirrhosis relationship, in that failure to take it into account generates a false picture. As already noted, it is precisely to avoid confounding that randomized studies are desirable. In nonrandomized studies of cardiovascular disease, where numerous and often intercorrelated risk factors exist, confounding is an important issue. To understand better how confounding works, consider the formula:

$$R_f = \frac{R_c P_1 + (1 - P_1)}{R_c P_2 + (1 - P_2)}$$

Here $R_c$ is the relative risk of disease resulting from exposure to the confounding variable, $P_1$ is the frequency of exposure to the confounder among people exposed to the agent of interest, and $P_2$ is the frequency among those not exposed. $R_f$ is the *apparent* relative risk in relation to the factor of interest, assuming that it is actually without effect on the disease. Examination of this formula allows four conclusions to be drawn: (1) If $R_c = 1$, $R_f = 1$. (2) If $P_1 = P_2$, $R_f = 1$. (3) Given $P_1$ and $P_2$, $R_f$ increases with $R_c$ reaching a maximum of $P_1/P_2$ when R is infinite. (4) Given $P_2$, the largest value of $R_f$ that can be achieved is $1/P_2$ when $P_1 = 1$ and $R_c$ is infinite.

Conclusions 1 and 2 limit the number of variables which need be given attention as potential confounding factors. Bias can only arise if a variable is associated *both* with risk of disease and with exposure to the agent.

Conclusions 3 and 4 affect the size of confounding effect that can arise from a particular variable. For a large bias to occur one needs the potential confounding variable to be relatively uncommon in those unexposed to the agent of interest and much more common in those exposed. In practice, therefore, confounding can relatively easily generate relative risks that are slightly greater than 1, but it requires special circumstances to explain a large relative risk. This is why strength of an association is so important in interpretation.

*Misclassification of Confounding Variables*

Often, statistical adjustment for a confounding variable reduces, but does not eliminate, the association of interest. Many workers assume, implicitly or explicitly, that if the association remains after adjustment then the confounding variable cannot fully explain the unadjusted association. This inference is only valid if the confounding variable is measured without error. When a confounder is measured inaccurately, adjustment will tend to be incomplete so that there will be an association remaining due to what is termed 'residual confounding'. A hypothetical example of this is shown in table 1. It is based on the following 6 assumptions: (1) An unobservable agent causes the disease, multiplying risk by 5 in those exposed. (2) The agent of interest does not in fact affect risk of disease. (3) 50% are exposed to the agent of interest. (4) 50% of those exposed to the agent of interest are exposed to the unobservable agent. (5) Exposure to the agent of interest and the unobservable agent are positively correlated. Thus 60% of those exposed to the unobservable agent are also exposed to the agent of interest. (6) The unobservable agent is inaccurately measured by the surrogate variable social class, with a 20% error in both directions.

The example shows the following typical results: (a) The strength of the relationship of disease with the surrogate variable social class (relative risk = 2.33) is less than that with the true but unobservable causal agent (RR = 5.00). (b) Confounding by the unobservable agent results in a spurious association (RR = 1.31) of the agent of interest with risk. (c) The spurious association with the agent of interest is not eliminated by adjusting for social class, the relative risk being 1.13 in low social class individuals, 1.33 in high social class individuals and 1.19 overall (using the Mantel-Haenszel [8] statistic to obtain an adjusted estimate).

A general conclusion is that one should be particularly wary in drawing conclusions where one knows the confounding variable is likely to be measured inaccurately and adjustment for it reduces but does not eliminate the association with the risk factor of interest. Apart from variables which are obvious surrogates for some difficult-to-measure true factor, such as social class (which does not of itself kill people, but may act as a marker for things that do), examples of confounding variables which are likely to be measured inaccurately are diet (people do not remember accurately what and how much they eat, especially in years gone by), and indices of sexual activity (which may be inaccurate markers of exposure to

*Table 1.* A hypothetical example of bias caused by misclassification of a confounding variable

| Subgroup(s) | Exposure to unobservable agent | Social class | Agent of interest | Number of subjects | Risk[1] |
|---|---|---|---|---|---|
| 1 | + | low | yes | 240 | 5 |
| 2 | + | low | no | 160 | 5 |
| 3 | + | high | yes | 60 | 5 |
| 4 | + | high | no | 40 | 5 |
| 5 | – | low | yes | 40 | 1 |
| 6 | – | low | no | 60 | 1 |
| 7 | – | high | yes | 160 | 1 |
| 8 | – | high | no | 240 | 1 |
| *Unadjusted effect of social class* | | | | | |
| 1 + 2 + 5 + 6 | | low | | 500 | 4.20 |
| 3 + 4 + 7 + 8 | | high | | 500 | 1.80 |
| | | | | | rr = 2.33 |
| *Unadjusted effect of agent of interest* | | | | | |
| 1 + 3 + 5 + 7 | | | yes | 500 | 3.40 |
| 2 + 4 + 6 + 8 | | | no | 500 | 2.60 |
| | | | | | rr = 1.31 |
| *Adjusted effect of agent of interest* | | | | | |
| (1) Among low social class | | | | | |
| 1 + 5 | | | yes | 280 | 4.43 |
| 2 + 6 | | | no | 220 | 3.91 |
| | | | | | rr = 1.13 |
| (2) Among high social class | | | | | |
| 3 + 7 | | | yes | 220 | 2.09 |
| 4 + 8 | | | no | 280 | 1.57 |
| | | | | | rr = 1.33 |

[1] Risks are relative to those not exposed to the unobservable agent. When subgroups are combined, risk is average per subject combined. rr = relative risk.

a sexually transmitted agent). Where there is a major risk factor which is inaccurately measured, it becomes very difficult, if not impossible, to come up with reliable evidence as to whether a weaker association seen with another factor, which is correlated with the major risk factor, is a true effect or is a result of confounding. A good example of this is the relationship of smoking to cervix cancer: it is known that risk of cervix cancer is strongly affected by a sexually transmitted agent (probably a virus), and that smokers have many more sexual partners than nonsmokers, and for this reason the multitude of reports of an association between smoking and cervix cancer are generally not treated as proof of a causal relationship.

A final point under this heading relates to misclassification which can arise due to an inappropriate statistical model. The use of multivariate logistic regression to adjust for confounding variables may sound impressive. However, it may lead to residual confounding not only if the confounding variables are inaccurately measured but also if false model assumptions of additivity of effect and linearity of dose-response relationships lead to the potential confounding effect of variables as measured not being fully accounted for.

*Misclassification of Exposure Status*

Where there is a major factor known to be very strongly associated with a disease and the effect of another minor factor is to be investigated, some researchers investigate the effect of the minor factor by restricting attention to those not exposed to the major factor. However, bias may still occur if the subjects are misclassified according to the major factor. A well-known example of this occurs when studying the relationship of various diseases to marriage to a smoker (as a marker of ETS exposure), where attention is restricted to those who are classified as never having smoked [9].

Generally this section and the previous one underline the difficulty in studying a weak association in the presence of an existing strong risk factor with which it is correlated.

*Dose Response*

It is important, where possible, to record not only whether a subject is exposed but also the degree (and duration) of exposure. Normally, a true relationship will be stronger with increasing exposure, and emphasis should be given to statistical tests that are powerful for the detection of such a dose-related trend. One should be cautious about accepting as evidence of a causal effect studies which show an association at low doses but not at high doses or which show a very irregular dose-response relationship. Even where the dose response does rise smoothly, a causal relationship must not be concluded too readily, since many of the mechanisms already discussed that produce bias in a simple association between a risk factor and disease will also produce a spurious dose-response relationship. Since heavy smoking and heavy drinking are strongly correlated, one would expect to see a dose-related relationship between smoking and liver cirrhosis even though there is no true effect.

*Effect of Stopping Exposure*

In some studies, evidence is available on individuals who were exposed to the risk factor of interest for a period, after which time exposure ceased. For acute effects, one would expect to see risk drop shortly after exposure to a level similar to that in the never exposed group, while for chronic effects one would expect to see a risk intermediate between that of those never exposed and those continuously exposed, with risk approaching that of those never exposed the longer the time after exposure stops. Evidence of patterns along these lines strengthens the argument that a causal relationship exists, though it must be pointed out that they might occur as a result of confounding. Evidence that risk is higher in those who cease exposure than in those who continue tends to cast doubt on the causal nature of an association, though it might not rule it out if presence of the disease makes people avoid exposure. It is interesting to note that though there is abundant evidence on risk in relation to stopping active smoking, there is little or no such data in relation to cessation of exposure to ETS.

*'Meta-Analysis' of Data from Multiple Studies*

It is widely accepted that data from small, similarly conducted, randomized trials may be combined in order to obtain a more accurate estimate of effect of exposure. Although meta-analyses are increasingly being conducted on data from observational studies, there are a number of doubts concerning the validity of such an approach. If the individual studies are open to the same source of bias (or even to different sources of bias) the overall estimate from the combined data will also be biassed. Even if the individual studies are unbiassed the overall estimate will only be unbiassed if the studies being combined are representative of all those that exist. However, it is amply documented that this is often not the case. Because scientists tend not to submit to journals, or journal editors tend not to publish, studies finding no association, or an association in an unexpected direction, the published evidence on many issues tends to overstate the real association. For some issues the overall association emerging from meta-analysis may be totally spurious.

The ideal way to avoid publication bias is to collect all the available data, but this is often difficult or impossible to achieve. In the absence of this, more weight might be given in meta-analysis to nonsignificant than to significant trials. In particular, the first published study might be given little or no weight as normally it generates the hypothesis so cannot be used to test it. Journals will, anyway, not usually accept a first study which shows no effect. Another, but more long-term, solution is to carry out 'quadruple blind studies'. As noted above, those defining disease status should be blind to the exposure, and those defining exposure should be blind to disease so as to avoid bias. To avoid nonreporting bias, one seems to require two further stages of blindness, in which both the scientist writing the paper and the journal refereeing it are blind to its results. The scientist would write two papers, each with a common introduction and methods section and with a common results section with identically structured tables but no data entered. Only the discussion section (and abstract) would vary, illustrating the different conclusions drawn by the author depending on whether or not a significant relationship was found. The journal would be sent both versions and must agree to accept both or neither. On acceptance, the data would be examined and the tables completed. Ideally, the journal would publish both discussion sections to show how the authors' opinion depended on the findings. This procedure not only eliminates publication bias, but also the possibility that authors select analyses to suit their beliefs.

In conclusion, the above should have given some insight into the main points to be taken into account when designing, analyzing and interpreting epidemiological studies. Perhaps the most important point is not to jump to conclusions too readily. An association, particularly a weak association, can arise as an artefact in so many ways in epidemiology that it is irresponsible to conclude cause and effect from an association without having carefully considered alternative explanations.

## *References*


1 Doll R, Peto R: Mortality in relation to smoking: 20 years' observations on male British doctors. Br Med J 1976;ii:1525–1536.

2 Cupples LA, D'Agostino RB: Section 34: Some risk factors related to the annual incidence of cardiovascular disease and death using pooled repeated biennial measurements: Framingham Heart Study, 30-year follow-up; in Kannel WB, Wolf PA, Garrison RJ (eds): The Framingham Study: An Epidemiological Investigation of Cardiovascular disease. NIH Publ No 87-2703. Washington, Department of Health and Human Services, 1987.

3 Carroll KK: Experimental evidence of dietary factors and hormone-dependent cancers. Cancer Res 1975;35:3374–3383.

4 Glantz S, Parmley W: Passive smoking and heart disease: Epidemiology, physiology and biochemistry. Circulation 1991;83:1–12.

5 Wells CK, Feinstein AR: Detection bias in diagnostic pursuit of lung cancer. Am J Epidemiol 1988;128:1016–1025.

6 Hirayama T: Cancer mortality in non-smoking women with smoking husbands based on a large-scale cohort study in Japan. Prev Med 1984;13:680–690.

7 Helsing KJ, Sandler DP, Comstock GW, Chu E: Heart disease mortality in non-smokers living with smokers. Am J Epidemiol 1988;127:915–922.

8 Mantel N, Haenszel W: Statistical aspects of the analysis of data from the retrospective study of disease. J Natl Cancer Inst 1959;22:719–748.
9 Lee PN: Misclassification of smoking habits and passive smoking. A review of the evidence. Int Arch Occup Environ Health, suppl. Berlin, Springer, 1988.

Peter N. Lee, MA, Consultant in Epidemiology and Statistics, 17 Cedar Road, Sutton, Surrey SM2 5DA (UK)

Weetman DF, Wood D (eds): Risk Factors for Cardiovascular Disease in Non-Smokers. Int. Workshop, Washington, Tyne and Wear, 1991. Basel, Karger, 1993, pp 86–94

# The Effect of Dietary Fat and Cholesterol on Plasma Total Cholesterol and Lipoprotein Cholesterol

*Andrew M. Salter*

Department of Applied Biochemistry and Food Science, University of Nottingham, Faculty of Agricultural and Food Sciences, Sutton Bonington, Loughborough, Leics., UK

A wealth of epidemiological evidence suggests that raised plasma cholesterol concentration represents a major risk factor for atherosclerotic vascular disease. More specifically it is elevated concentrations of cholesterol in the low density lipoprotein (LDL) fraction that are most strongly related to increased risk. Conversely, high levels of high density lipoprotein (HDL) cholesterol appear to be protective from the disease. The concentration of cholesterol in the plasma and its distribution between different lipoprotein fractions is regulated by a range of genetic, metabolic and dietary factors. Two of the most studied dietary influences are the amount of dietary cholesterol consumed and the quantity and type of dietary fat. The aim of this review is to present a brief overview of our current understanding of the effects of dietary cholesterol and fat on plasma lipoprotein cholesterol concentrations.

## *Dietary Cholesterol*

The cholesterol content of the body represents a balance between synthesis (primarily in the liver), dietary consumption, metabolism and excretion. Cholesterol synthesis in humans represents something like 1,000 mg/day which is considerably more than is normally consumed in the diet. In the normal Western diet, eggs represent the major source of dietary cholesterol with a medium size egg (50 g) yielding about 200 mg. While certain other foods, including butter, liver and shrimps, contain relatively high concentrations, these are not normally regularly consumed in any great quantity. Plant material is free of cholesterol and levels in meat and animal fat are fairly low.

The extent to which dietary cholesterol can affect plasma cholesterol concentrations remains controversial. Studies on a number of species of laboratory animals have shown that feeding large amounts of cholesterol results in marked hypercholesterolaemia and the development of atherosclerosis. However, demonstrating a direct relationship between more modest cholesterol consumption and plasma cholesterol concentrations within human populations has proven difficult. One major reason for this is that the contents of saturated fat and cholesterol within a diet tend to be highly correlated. Thus on a population basis it is difficult to attribute specific differences in plasma cholesterol to dietary cholesterol alone.

The most persuasive evidence for a relationship between cholesterol in the diet and the plasma comes from feeding studies. In the mid-1960s, Keys and co-workers [1] attempted to quantify the effect of dietary cholesterol on plasma cholesterol by bringing together a number of cholesterol feeding experiments and correlating the change in plasma cholesterol with the amount consumed. His results can be summarized in the following equation:

$$\triangle \text{chol} = 1.5(Z_1 - Z_2)$$

where $\triangle$chol = change in plasma cholesterol (mg/dl); $Z_2$ = the square root of the new cholesterol intake (mg/1,000 kcal); $Z_1$ = the square root of the initial cholesterol intake (mg/1,000 kcal).

One of the most significant aspects of this equation is that the change in plasma cholesterol is related to the square root of the change in dietary cholesterol. This means that even quite large changes in dietary cholesterol intake result in only modest changes in plasma concentrations. For example, if a man consuming 3,000 kcal/day were to increase his consumption of eggs from 1 to 3, and this represented the only source of dietary cholesterol, then his plasma cholesterol would only rise by 9 mg/dl. At a normal plasma cholesterol level of about 200 mg/dl this would represent a rise of less than 5%. Thus, for the vast majority of individuals, who probably consume less than 2 eggs per day, dietary cholesterol intake in itself probably has little effect on cholesterol homeostasis, especially as increases in dietary intake are normally compensated for by a decrease in hepatic cholesterol synthesis.

On a population basis, the Keys equation is a fairly good description of the effect of dietary cholesterol on plasma levels. In 1984, Keys [2] re-evaluated the formula and showed that it predicted quite well the results of a further 20 feeding trials which had been performed since it was originally published.

Two major limitations of the Keys equation are that it does not predict changes in individual lipoprotein fractions and it does not account for individual variations in response. In a review of 10 recent studies, Beynen and Katan [3] show that in all but one study increasing dietary cholesterol increased total serum cholesterol. In terms of the individual lipoprotein fractions, LDL cholesterol was measured in 8 of the 10 studies and was found to increase with the amount of cholesterol consumed. They concluded that about 85% of the increase in total plasma cholesterol could be attributed to the LDL fraction. The effect of dietary cholesterol on HDL cholesterol was more variable, with 6 of the studies showing an increase, 3 a decrease and 1 no change.

The question of individual responses to dietary cholesterol has been the subject of considerable research. In many studies significant variation in the response to dietary cholesterol has been noted between individuals. This has led to the concept of hypo- and hyperresponders. While a certain amount of this variation should be attributed to nonreproducible chance fluctuations [4], there do appear to be individuals within the population who do not respond in the same way as the majority. It has recently been suggested that this may be genetically linked to the occurrence of different phenotypes of apolipoprotein (apo) E [5]. This protein is an important component of many plasma lipoproteins, especially chylomicrons, which carry dietary fats and cholesterol. Plasma cholesterol many increase to a greater extent, in response to dietary cholesterol, in those carrying the apo E4 phenotype compared to those carrying apo E2, with apo E3 being intermediate. Thus, those individuals who are homozygous for apo E4 may be hyperresponders while apo E2 homozygotes may be hyporesponders.

### *Dietary Fat*

In a similar way to his analysis of dietary cholesterol, Keys [6] has produced an equation that predicts the effect of changes in dietary fat on plasma cholesterol concentrations:

$$\triangle \text{chol} = 1.2(2\triangle S - \triangle P)$$

where $\triangle$chol = change in plasma cholesterol (mg/dl), and $\triangle S$ and $\triangle P$ represent the change in the percentage of total calories supplied as glycerides of saturated and polyunsaturated fatty acids respectively.

The major point to note in this equation is that saturated fat is twice as effective at raising plasma cholesterol as polyunsaturated fat is at lowering it.

Keys [6] recognized that some saturated fatty acids are more potent at increasing plasma cholesterol than others. In general, those that fit the equation best are the medium chain fatty acids: lauric (C12:0), myristic (C14:0) and palmitic (C16:0). All are found in abundance in some plant oils such as coconut and palm kernel oil while the latter represents a major component of most animal fats. Stearic acid (C18:0), a major component of cocoa butter as well as most animal fats, is a notable exception to the Keys equation. A number of studies have shown it not to raise plasma cholesterol [6–9]. However, these studies used natural sources of the acid and some evidence exists to suggest that, in its pure form, stearic acid may be as hypercholesterolaemic as palmitic acid [10]. The effect of this particular fatty acid deserves further consideration as it could be potentially useful in the food industry because, as a saturated fatty acid, it is solid at room temperature. Thus, it could be incorporated into fat blends, such as margarines, replacing hydrogenation processes currently used to 'harden' such fats: these processes can produce potentially harmful 'trans' fatty acids (see below).

Polyunsaturated fats exist in two major forms; the n – 6 type and the n – 3 type (this refers to the position of the first double bond in the carbon chain). The most common n – 6 fatty acid is linoleic acid (C18:2) which is often the predominant fatty acid in certain strains of sunflower and rape seed oil. Much smaller quantities of γ-linolenic acid (C18:3) are also present in the diet. The major dietary n – 3 fatty acid of most non-coastal populations is α-linolenic acid also found in vegetable oils. However, fat derived from fish and marine mammals is enriched in longer chain n – 3 fatty acids, predominantly eicosapentaenoic acid (EPA, C20:5) and docosahexaenoic acid (DHA, C22:6). Thus, for most dietary fat sources the major polyunsaturated fatty acid is linoleic acid and it is for this that the Keys equation is really designed.

The effects of γ- and α-linolenic acid on plasma cholesterol have been subject to only a limited amount of study. Some [11], but not all [12], workers have demonstrated a hypocholesterolaemic effect of evening primrose oil, which is particularly rich in linolenic acid. In a study comparing the effects of sunflower oil and linseed oil (rich in linoleic and α-linolenic acids respectively) the cholesterol-lowering ability of both appeared to be about equal [13].

The low incidence of heart disease and low plasma lipid concentrations in a number of coastal populations, such as Greenland Eskimos [14, 15], has led to a great deal of interest in the possible benefits of diets enriched in the marine fatty acids. Much controversy still remains over their effect on plasma cholesterol concentrations. This subject has recently been reviewed in considerable detail by Harris [16]. Early studies using large doses of fish oil apparently showed them to be effective at lowering both plasma cholesterol and triacylglycerol concentrations. More recent, better controlled studies, with more moderate amounts of fish oil, have tended to confirm their hypotriglyceridaemic effect but not that on plasma cholesterol. Thus, current evidence suggests that the amount of fish oil that would be required to reduce plasma cholesterol concentrations would be impractical for the vast majority of people. However, there may be other possible beneficial effects of fish oil on other risk factors for heart disease, such as platelet function, blood pressure and perhaps plasma triacylglycerol, the status of which as an independent risk factor still remains uncertain.

When Keys formulated his equation, the effect of monounsaturated fatty acids was assumed to be neutral, i.e. similar to an equivalent amount of carbohydrate, and was therefore not included. Oleic acid (cis C18 : 1), which is found throughout the animal and plant kingdom, is the most abundant monounsaturate in the diet and its status as 'neutral' has recently been challenged. Some workers [17] have suggested that not only may it be almost as potent as linoleic acid in reducing total plasma cholesterol, but it may also produce a more favourable plasma lipoprotein profile (see below). One reason why Mediterranean populations have a relatively low incidence of heart disease may be the consumption of large quantities of olive oil, which is oleic acid-rich.

The trans-isomer of oleic acid, elaidic acid, whilst less common in the plant and animal kingdoms, does occur in considerable quantities in fats which have undergone hydrogenation, both biologically, in ruminants, and during hardening for the production of solid margarines and vegetable oils, Recent studies suggest that, relative to oleic acid, they may raise plasma cholesterol [18]. If this proves to be correct then consideration should be given to developing new ways of hardening vegetable oils.

In general, increasing the ratio of polyunsaturated to saturated (P/S ratio) fat in the diet reduces LDL cholesterol. However, the effect on HDL cholesterol appears to be much more variable, with most studies showing decreased levels, but some showing unchanged or even increased levels [3]. Oleic acid appears to decrease LDL cholesterol concentrations without affecting HDL. Thus, if polyunsaturates really do reduce HDL concentrations, then this may suggest a major benefit of monounsaturates. Coupled with the other health-associated problems that may be correlated with high intakes of polyunsaturates, such as increased risk of cancer [19], the conventional advice of replacing saturated fat in the diet with polyunsaturates should perhaps be reconsidered in favour of oleic acid. Elaidic acid, unlike its isomer, appears to have a specific effect in lowering plasma HDL while increasing LDL [18]. This is again evidence that it may be desirable to remove elaidic acid from the diet. As with total cholesterol, moderate consumption of fish oils appears to have little effect on the cholesterol concentration of either LDL or HDL [16]. In fact, in hypertriglyceridaemic patients, fish oils have been shown actually to increase LDL cholesterol concentrations.

As with dietary cholesterol, it has been suggested that certain individuals may be hyperresponsive to the cholesterol-raising effects of saturated fat. In fact, the same individuals may be hyperresponsive to both these dietary parameters [20].

### *Reducing Total Fat Consumption*

In general, modern dietary recommendations for reducing risk of developing premature heart disease include reducing both the total amount of fat consumed as well as the proportion of that fat which is saturated. Unless you are to reduce the total calorie intake, which in many cases could in itself be beneficial, then fat excluded from the diet has to be replaced with other nutrients, usually carbohydrate. The Keys equation regards carbohydrate and oleic acid as having similar 'neutral' effects on total plasma cholesterol and most subsequent investigations have supported this. However, some evidence exists to suggest that high carbohydrate/low fat diets may produce lipoprotein profiles that may actually be unfavourable. In general, displacing fat with carbohydrate tends to reduce HDL more consistently than LDL cholesterol [3]. This effect on HDL suggests that a potentially more protective lipoprotein profile would be gained by substituting saturated fat with oleic acid rather than with carbohydrate.

In conclusion, despite the vast amount of research that has been performed in humans and animals, the exact role of dietary cholesterol and fat in regulating plasma lipoprotein cholesterol concentration still remains unclear. The present consensus of opinion is that, in the majority of people, dietary cholesterol has little effect on plasma lipoprotein cholesterol concentration. However, there may be certain individuals who are more responsive and an increased effort to identify these people may be more productive than recommending a reduction in cholesterol consumption for the whole population.

Table 1 attempts to summarize the effect of different dietary fatty acids on total plasma cholesterol and lipoprotein cholesterol. It should be recognized that the evidence for the effect of some of these fatty acids is much stronger than that for others. In general, saturated fatty acids in the diet appear to be a major factor in influencing plasma cholesterol levels and its major effect seems to be on the atherogenic LDL fraction. However, what we should replace this with in the diet remains unclear. While some reduction in total fat consumption would seem prudent, replacing large

*Table 1.* Summary of the effect of dietary fatty acids on plasma total and lipoprotein cholesterol concentrations

| Fatty acid | Formula | Total cholesterol | LDL cholesterol | HDL cholesterol |
|---|---|---|---|---|
| Lauric | C12:0 | + + + | + + + | + |
| Myristic | C14:0 | + + + | + + + | + |
| Palmitic | C16:0 | + + + | + + + | + |
| Stearic | C18:0 | 0 | 0 | 0 |
| Oleic | C18:1 cis | – | – | 0 |
| Elaidic | C18:1 trans | + | + + | – |
| Linoleic | C18:2 | – – | – – | – |
| γ-Linolenic | C18:3 (n – 6) | – – | – – | – |
| α-Linolenic | C18:3 (n – 3) | – – | – – | – |
| Eicosapentaenoic | C20:5 (n – 3) | 0 | 0 | 0 |
| Docosahexaenoic | C22:6 (n – 3) | 0 | 0 | 0 |

+ = Increase; – = decrease; 0 = no effect. Number of symbols indicates potency of effect.

amounts of fat with carbohydrate may well have the adverse effect of reducing the protective HDL cholesterol fraction.

Substituting saturated fat with either linoleic or oleic acid appears to reduce plasma LDL but the polyunsaturated fatty acid does this at the expense of reducing HDL cholesterol as well. n – 3 polyunsaturated fatty acids of marine origin appear to have little beneficial effect on lipoprotein cholesterol levels. Thus, our present knowledge suggests that replacement of saturated fat with monounsaturated fat in the diet may be the best way to reduce our plasma LDL cholesterol concentrations, thereby decreasing the risk of developing premature atherosclerotic vascular disease. However, this still remains to be proven in well-designed, well-executed, human feeding trials.

## *References*


1 Grande F, Anderson JT, Chouverakis C, Proja M, Keys A: Effects of dietary cholesterol on man's serum lipids, J Nutr 1965;87:52–62.

2 Keys A: Serum cholesterol response to dietary cholesterol. Am J Clin Nutr 1984;40: 351–359.

3 Beynen AC, Katan MB: Impact of dietary cholesterol and fatty acids on serum lipids and lipoproteins in man; in Vergroessen AJ, Crawford M (eds): The role of Fats in Human Nutrition. London, Academic Press, 1989, pp 237–286.

4 Beynen AC, Katan MB: Reproducibility of individual serum cholesterol response to diet. Am J Clin Nutr 1988;48:1518–1520.

5 Miettinen TA, Kesaniemi TA: Cholesterol absorption regulates cholesterol metabolism and within-population variation of serum cholesterol; in Suckling KE, Groot PHE (eds): Hyperlipidaemia and Atherosclerosis. London, Academic Press, 1988, pp 73–82.
6 Keys A, Anderson JT, Grande F: Serum cholesterol response to changes in diet. IV. Particular saturated fatty acids in the diet. Metabolism 1965;14:776–787.
7 Hegsted DM, McGandy RB, Myers ML, Store FJ: Quantitiative effects of dietary fat on serum cholesterol in man. Am J Clin Nutr 1965;17:281–295.
8 Grande F, Anderson JT, Keys A: Comparison of effects of palmitic and stearic acids in the diet on serum cholesterol in man. Am J Clin Nutr 1970;23:1184–1193.
9 Bonanome A, Grundy SM: Effects of dietary stearic acid on plasma cholesterol and lipoprotein levels. N Engl J Med 1988;318:1244–1248.
10 McGandy RB, Hegsted DM, Myer ML: Use of semi-synthetic fats in determining effects of specific dietary fatty acids on serum lipids in man. Am J Clin Nutr 1970;23:1288–1298.
11 Horrobin DF, Manku MS: How do polyunsaturated fatty acids lower plasma cholesterol levels? Lipids 1983;18:588–592.
12 Boberg M, Vessby B, Selinus I: Effect of dietary supplementation with n – 6 and n – 3 long-chain polyunsaturated fatty acids on serum lipoproteins and platelet function in hypertriglyceridaemic patients. Acta Med Scand 1986;220:153–160.
13 Singer P, Berger I, Wirth M, Godicke W, Jaeger W, Voigt S: Slow desaturation and elongation of linoleic and α-linolenic acids as a rationale of eicosapentaenic acid-rich diet to lower blood pressure and serum lipids in normal, hypertensive and hyperlipidaemic subjects. Prostaglandins Leukot Med 1986;24:173–193.
14 Kromann N, Green A: Epidemiological studies in the Upernavik district, Greenland. Incidence of some chronic diseases 1950–1974. Acta Med Scand 1980;208:401–406.
15 Dyerberg J, Jorgensen KA: Marine oils and thrombogenesis. Prog Lipid Res 1982;21:255–269.
16 Harris WS: Fish oils and plasma lipid and lipoprotein metabolism in humans: A critical review. J Lipid Res 1989;30:785–807.
17 Grundy SM, Denke MA: Dietary influences on serum lipids and lipoproteins. J Lipid Res 1990;31:1149–1172.
18 Mensink RP, Katan MB: Effect of dietary trans fatty acids on high-density and low-density lipoprotein cholesterol levels in healthy subjects. N Engl J Med 1990; 323:439–441.
19 Vergroesen AJ: Introduction: in Vergroessen AJ, Crawford M (eds): The Role of Fats in Human Nutrition. London, Academic Press, 1989, pp 5–36.
20 Katan MB, Berns MAM, Glatz JFC, Knuiman JT, Nobels A, DeVries JHM: Congruence of individual responsiveness to dietary cholesterol and to saturated fat in man. J Lipid Res 1988;29:883–892.


A.M. Salter, MD, Department of Applied Biochemistry and Food Science, University of Nottingham, Faculty of Agricultural and Food Sciences, Sutton Bonington, Loughborough, Leicestershire LE12 5RD (UK)

## *Discussion*

*Bruckdorfer* (London): It's interesting how fashions have changed. In the early 60s, Aarons produced some data showing the beneficial effects of monounsaturates and the lack of effect or neutral effects of stearic acid. I think the scientific world chose to ignore those results until they were resurrected by Scott Grundy 20 years later. And now there are suggestions that in animal experiments, polyunsaturates might actually be immunosuppressive if taken in the bulk of something like 12% of the diet. There is no human experience of having very high polyunsaturated fatty acids in the diets, but there is plenty with monounsaturates, so I think there is common sense in what you're saying: Looking to the monounsaturates as being the major constituent of fat in the diet if we've got to have fat at all.

*Salter* (Nottingham): I agree with you completely.

*Gardiner* (Airdrie): Can I ask how C18:0 could be introduced into the diet?

*Salter*: Things like cocoa butter are rich in C18:0, but it is being suggested that the food industry should look at the biological activity of the fats that they're producing, and rather than pushing the polyunsaturated fats relentlessly, they should be trying to introduce C18:0 into some foods, particularly into the margarines which you want hard. C18:0 is an ideal hardener for fat, rather than hydrogenation which might produce trans-C18:1 which might be hypercholesterolaemic.

*Bruckdorfer*: I just wondered if you could comment on the fact that Masai people in East Africa have a very high cholesterol intake and yet have low plasma cholesterol levels – What do you think the explanation for that is?

*Salter*: I don't know. The effect of dietary cholesterol is probably very weak. Going to populations which are essentially cholesterol-free will probably identify people who have particularly low plasma cholesterol. Increasing dietary cholesterol probably doesn't have an equal effect in increasing it in the plasma.

Weetman DF, Wood D (eds): Risk Factors for Cardiovascular Disease in Non-Smokers. Int. Workshop, Washington, Tyne and Wear, 1991. Basel, Karger, 1993, pp 95–99

# Exercise: Protection or Provocation?

*Peter A. Butlin*

Northern Institute for Sport Science and Exercise Medicine,
School of Health Sciences, University of Sunderland, UK

Results of various epidemiological studies have shown that men involved in moderate to vigorous levels of physical activity were less at risk for cardiovascular disease than were those rated as inactive [1–9]. Women are less at risk for cardiovascular diseases than men, and there is inadequate evidence to decide if they benefit from exercise in the way that men do [10].

Physical activity has been shown to counteract known risk factors for cardiovascular disease. As indicated below, regular exercise can produce the following changes: (a) reduction of systolic and diastolic arterial blood pressure [11–13]; (b) an increase in high-density lipoprotein cholesterol and a reduction in low-density lipoprotein cholesterol levels in the blood [14, 15]; (c) a decrease in the processes of blood clotting and platelet aggregation [8, 16, 17] and (d) a reduction in body weight and the prevention of weight gain [18].

It is believed that the relative risk of physical inactivity may be far greater than has previously been accepted, and may approach the relative risks usually attributed to cigarette smoking, hypertension and hypercholesterolaemia (table 1) [19, 20].

In order to promote physical activity, there has been a great deal of literature advocating exercise, which usually prescribes regimens of brisk activity for a period of 15–30 min duration, 2–3 times/week [21–24].

The research findings that have led to the recommendation of this level of exercise are based on aerobic fitness, signified by increases in maximal oxygen uptake. However, few epidemiological studies have shown any evidence for an increase in aerobic fitness to be an indicator of a reduced risk in cardiovascular disease [25]. It may be that the level of exercise that has been advocated for improving aerobic fitness is not necessarily the same as that which reduces the risk of cardiovascular disease.

*Table 1.* Comparison of the relative risks for cardiovascular diseases from physical inactivity relative to some other factors

| | Relative risk |
|---|---|
| Physical inactivity in men | 1.9–2.4 |
| Smoking 20 cigarettes/day | 2.5 |
| Hypertension | 2.1 |
| Hypercholesterolaemia | 2.4 [19, 20] |

This raises two important questions for those who advocate increasing physical activity levels: (1) Is the term 'exercise' suitable for use within heathy life-style programmes? (2) Is continuous physical activity recommended to improve a level of aerobic fitness, prescribed as 2–3 times/week in bouts of 15–30 min duration, a realistic goal of achievement for many people?

Before one should advocate the incorporation of a programme of physical activity into any individual's life-style programme, information relating to these questions should be known and clearly understood.

Exercise is a term often synonymous with sporting activity. The term 'to take exercise' implies that one should perform a physical act distinct from the normal daily routine. For many people, this means implementing an additional unfamiliar activity, such as jogging.

Health problems associated with sporting activities include injuries to joints, tendon and muscles and, in extreme cases sudden death, presumably from myocardial infarction [26, 27]. Many people taking exercise, or about to participate in an exercise programme, will be deterred by such reports in the media as that which occurred when James Fixx, the author of one of America's best-selling books on running [28], collapsed and died whilst out on his daily run. However, for many people, sporting activity is enjoyable. It brings people together, relieves the stresses and tensions of work and provides an outlet for physical activity which is beyond that of a normal daily routine. For these reasons, sport can be regarded as a healthy pastime and should be encouraged within prescribed activity programmes.

For those who are resistant to the ethos surrounding exercise, a realistic target is an increase in energy expenditure. Results of studies carried out by Morris *et al.* [7] and Chave *et al.* [29] showed that the risk of cardiovascular disease was less in people who reported vigorous activity in their leisure time. The measure of vigorous activity was defined as a peak energy expenditure greater than 7.5 kcal/min. Paffenbarger *et al.* [6,

30] showed that the risk of cardiovascular disease declined in those people with an additional weekly energy expenditure of 2,000 kcal and that little benefit was gained from values above this figure. Such level of activity can quite easily be obtained by a brisk walking program, stair climbing or gardening activities. It does not necessarily have to include the prescribed amounts of aerobic activity which is advocated to maintain cardiovascular fitness levels.

The middle-aged male, the elderly, the disabled, the obese, and those with a low socioeconomic status are generally identified as being at a high risk for cardiovascular disease. For many of these people an involvement in exercise programmes designed to achieve the optimal level of aerobic fitness would be quite unrealistic. It has been shown that it is unlikely that their introduction to such an exercise programme would result in their life-long compliance with the activity.

Oldridge [31] has shown that only a small percentage of people embarking on an aerobic training programme will continue after 3 years. Therefore, it would appear that, in line with the epidemiological evidence, the risk of cardiovascular disease is just as likely to decline from an increase in physical activity, irrespective of whether or not it is aerobic. In practical terms, this means that healthy life-style programmes that advocate an increase in physical activity may include sport and exercise for some individuals; however, they should also include sensible ways of increasing daily energy expenditure for all people. Those who recommend the use of exercise must consider the groups most at risk from cardiovascular disease. These people should be helped to make physical activity enjoyable, cheap and a part of their natural habitual activity. Some forms of exercise are harmful and detrimental to the promotion of good health, but the benefits which accrue from natural physical activity far outweigh the risks which people take in exercising.

## *References*

1 Froelicher VF, Brown P: Exercise and coronary heart disease. J Cardiovasc Rehabil 1981(Sept):227–288.

2 Leon AS, Blackburn H: The relationship of physical activity to coronary heart disease and life expectancy. Ann NY Acad Sci 1977;301:561–578.

3 Wyndham CH: The role of physical activity in the prevention of ischaemic heart disease: A review. S Afr Med J 1979;56:7–13.

4 Morris JN, Heady JA, Raffle PAB, Roberts CG, Epstein L, Sheehan DS: Coronary heart disease and physical activity of work. Lancet 1953;ii:1053–1057, 1111–1120.

5 Paffenbarger RS, Hole WE: Work activity and coronary heart mortality. N Engl J Med 1975;292:545–550.

6 Paffenbarger RS, Wing AL, Hyde RT: Physical activity as an index of heart attack risk in college alumni. Am J Epidemiol 1978;108:161–175.
7 Morris JN, Everitt MG, Pollard R, Chave SPW: Vigorous exercise in leisure time: Protection against coronary heart disease. Lancet 1980;ii:1207–1210.
8 Morris JN, Clayton DG, Everitt MG, Semmence AM, Burgess EH: Exercise in leisure time: Coronary attack and death dates. Br Heart J 1990;63:325–334.
9 Paffenbarger RS, Hydem RT, Wing AL, Hsieh C: Physical activity, all-cause mortality and longevity of college alumni. N Engl J Med 1986;314:605–613.
10 Hardman A: Exercise and the Heart: Report of a British Heart Foundation Working Group. 1991, p. 2.
11 Cade R, Mars D, Wagemaker H, Zouner C, Packer D, Privette M, Cade M, Peterson J, Hood-Lewis D. Effect of aerobic exercise training on patients with systemic arterial hypertension. Am J Med 1984;77:785–790.
12 Duncan JJ, Farr JE, Upton SJ, Hagan RD, Oglesby ME, Blair SN: The effects of aerobic exercise on plasma catecholamines and blood pressure in patients with mild essential hypertension. JAMA 1985;254:2609–2613.
13 Nelson L, Jennings GL, Ecler MD, Komer PI: Effect of changing levels of physical inactivity on blood pressure and haemodynamics in essential hypertension. Lancet 1986;ii:473–476.
14 Brownell KD, Bachorik PS, Ayerkem RS: Changes in plasma lipid and lipoprotein levels in men and women after a programme of moderate exercise. Circulation 1982;65:477–484.
15 Hardman AE, Hudson J, Jones PRM, Norgan NG: Brisk walking and high density lipoprotein cholesterol concentration in formerly sedentary women. Br Med J 1989;199:1204–1205.
16 Andrew M, Carter C, O'Brodovich H, Heigenhauser G: Increases in factor VIII complex and fibrinolytic activity are dependent on exercise intensity. J Appl Physiol 1986;60:1917–1922.
17 Ferguson EW, Bernier LL, Barton GR, Yu-Yehiro J, Schoomaker EB: Effects of exercise and conditioning on clotting and fibrinolytic activity in men. J Appl Physiol 1987;62:1416–1421.
18 Wood PD, Haskell WL, Blair SN, Williams PT, Krauss RN, Lingren FT, Albers JJ, Ho PH, Farquhar JW: Increased exercise level and plasma lipoprotein concentrations: A one-year, randomised, controlled study in sedentary, middle-aged men. Metabolism 1983;32:31–39.
19 Powell KE, Thompson PD, Casperson CJ, Kendrick JS: Physical activity and the incidence of coronary heart disease. Annu Rev Public Health 1987;8:253–287.
20 Pooling Project Research Group: Relationship of blood pressure, serum cholesterol, smoking habit, relative weight and ECG abnormalities to incidence of major coronary events: Final report of the Pooling Project. J Chronic Dis 1978;31:202–306.
21 Bassey EJ, Fentem PH: Exercise the Facts. Oxford, Oxford University Press, 1981.
22 Ashton D, Davies B. Why Exercise? Oxford, Blackwell, 1986.
23 The Coronary Prevention Group: Exercise Heart Health. The Coronary Prevention Group, 1987.
24 Fentem PH, Bassey EJ, Turnbull NB: The New Case for Exercise. London, Health Education Authority and the Sports Council, 1988.
25 La Porte RE, Dearwater S, Cauley JA, Slemenda C, Cook T: Cardiovascular fitness: Is it really necessary? Physician Sportsmed 1985;3:145–150.
26 Geiringer E: Sport as a threat to physical and mental health. NZ J Health, Physical Educ Recreation 1971;4:19–27.

27 Opie LH: Sudden death and sport. Lancet 1975;i:263–266.
28 Fixx J: The Complete Book of Running. London, Chatto & Windus, 1979.
29 Chave SPW, Morris JN, Mass S: Vigorous exercise in leisure-time: Protection against coronary heart disease, J Epidemiol Community Health 1978;32:239–243.
30 Paffenbarger RS Jr, Hyde RT, Wing AL: A natural history of athletics and cardiovascular health. JAMA 1984;252:491–495.
31 Oldridge NB: Compliance and exercise in primary and secondary prevention of coronary heart disease: a review. Prev Med 1982;II(January):56–70.

Peter Anthony Butlin, Northern Institute for Sport Science and Exercise Medicine,
School of Health Sciences, University of Sunderland,
Sunderland, Tyne and Wear SR1 3SD (UK)

Weetman DF, Wood D (eds): Risk Factors for Cardiovascular Disease in Non-Smokers. Int. Workshop, Washington, Tyne and Wear, 1991. Basel, Karger, 1993, pp 100–107

# Stress at Work and Cardiovascular Disease

*Lars Werko*

The Swedish Council on Technology Assessment in Health Care, Stockholm, Sweden

In the many epidemiological studies on ischaemic heart disease that have been conducted since World War II, the main emphasis has been on the so-called risk factors of high blood pressure, elevated blood lipids and cigarette smoking. These three factors have been designated as 'classical risk markers' for coronary heart disease. However, their presence in a middle-aged male population does not explain or account for more than about 50% of the ensuing cases of ischaemic or coronary heart disease [1] and there is thus ample room for other influences to be of importance. If you ask anyone in the population what factors they consider to be of great importance in the development of premature heart disease, the most frequent answer would be that stress must be one of the most important factors. Usually no definition of stress is then given, as this expression is thought to be self-explanatory.

## *A Model to Analyse Stress in the Work Environment*

The scientific study of stress started early this century and was accelerated in the 1940s–50s when Hans Selye [2], using this expression in animal experiments, demonstrated that nervous and hormonal influences led to the development of various diseases and especially cardiovascular disorders. Selye's work pointed to the important connections between higher nervous centres, mid-brain, endocrine glands and the cardiovascular system. His definition of stress was, however, not sufficiently detailed and circumscribed, nor was it precise enough to be used in daily clinical work. The early researchers in the field of psychosomatic medicine thus had difficulties in using this concept of stress, and the expression lost its scientific value for a time. In the meantime, neurophysiologists further explored the connections between the mid-brain and the visceral and

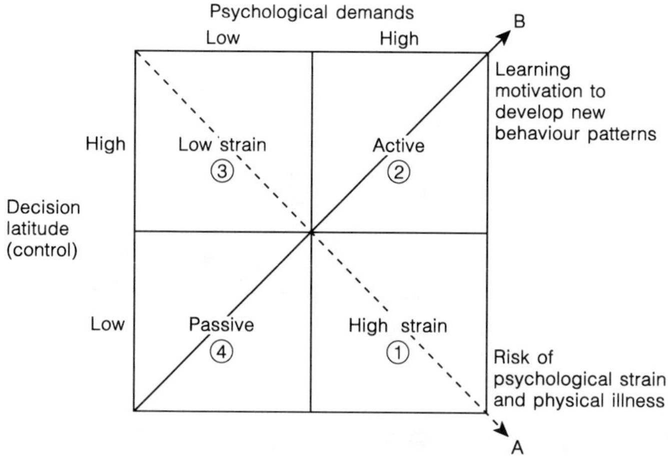


*Fig. 1.* Psychological demand/decision latitude model [data from 4].

cardiovascular systems. They were able to demonstrate the importance of signals from the brain for symptoms such as tachycardia, increased blood pressure and acceleration of intestinal motility during fear, anxiety or other situations when the individual felt himself threatened by occurrences in the environment.

However, it was not until Robert Karasek, in several publications alone or together with Tores Theorell [3], explored his concept of stress in the work environment that a practically useful definition of stress was introduced. These workers contrasted the demand exercised on the individual during work with his or her ability to influence the situation (decision latitude). Stress with pathophysiological consequences to the individual occurred only when high demands were combined in situations where the individual had no or very little opportunity to modify the work environment, in respect of physical background, strict time frames, personal contacts or other circumstances that might induce negative feelings in the individual (fig. 1). The difference between the executive in a demanding position but with complete freedom to arrange how the work is conducted, and the assembly worker situated at the assembly line performing the same routine, often pressed for time, throughout the working day, is obvious.

Karasek has grouped different types of work in relation to psychological demands and decision latitude, based on a large survey (fig. 2). Karasek and Theorell, with various co-workers [5, 6] have tried to evaluate their concept in several investigations comprising different categories of workers, and in prospective studies with special emphasis on the occurrence

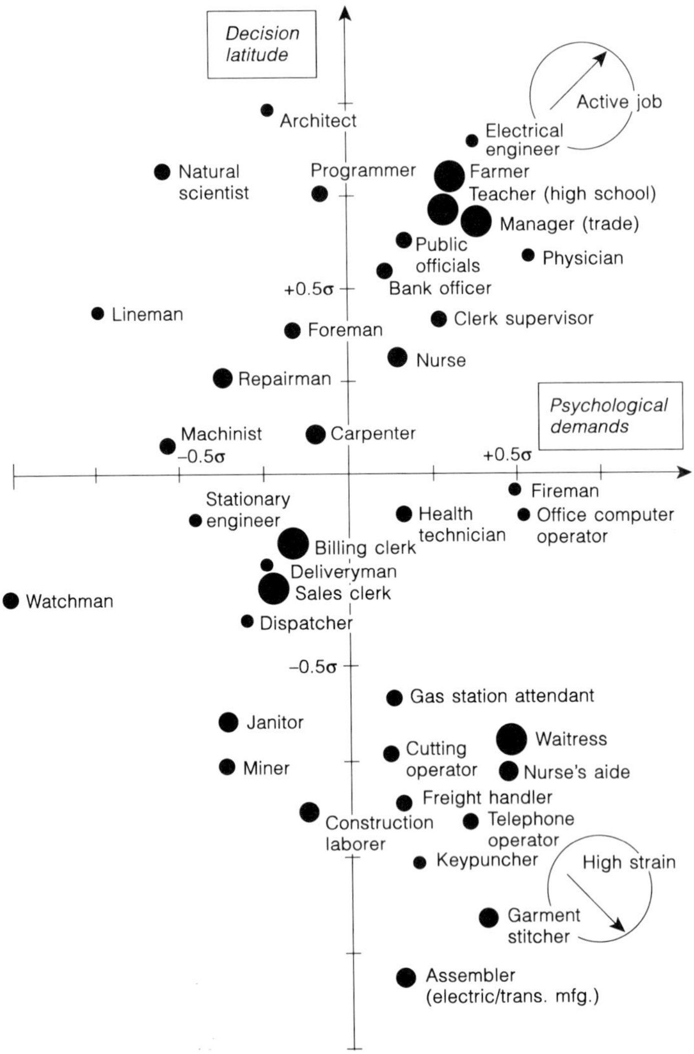


*Fig. 2.* The occupational distribution of psychological demands and decision latitude (US males and females, n = 4,495) [data from 4].

of cardiovascular disease. Thus, in large retrospectively studied series, they have found increased cardiovascular mortality or morbidity in occupations characterized by increased demands but with low degree of influence. Also, in smaller prospective case-control studies, they have been able to demonstrate the validity of this definition of 'job strain'. In these studies the characteristics of work were related to hospitalization for cardiovascular disorders, to subjective symptoms or to the occurrence of raised blood pressure. In some series this definition of 'job strain' has been related to symptoms such as lack of sleep, acute increases in heart rate and blood pressure, decreased feeling of well-being or changes in excretion of hormones.

Most of these investigations have, however, only considered the situation at work and have more or less neglected other factors of importance for the development of symptoms or signs of cardiovascular disease. More studies are thus needed where other risk factors, and especially the classic ones, are determined simultaneously with the analysis of the situation at the work site. The well-known effect of belonging to a defined social class must also be taken into account. This is important since the types of occupations where the job strain as defined by Karasek is high are often, but not always, combined with a lower social class. One important task for future investigations is thus to sort out the influence of social class from the effect of job strain, when judging the relative importance of these two factors for the development of severe cardiovascular disease.

### *Stress and the Cardiovascular System*

In a recent review of the literature on cardiovascular diseases and the work environment, Kristensen [7] concluded that the Karasek hypothesis has been strongly confirmed by several studies published in the epidemiological literature up to 1989. In a number of these studies, high or elevated blood pressure, rather than any definite diagnosis of cardiovascular damage, was used as a sign of cardiovascular involvement. In this context it is important to note that increase of blood pressure on physical and physiological stress may be a normal response, provided it is not excessive or long-lasting. One of the difficulties in explaining the connection between psyche, brain metabolism or brain transmitters and the cardiovascular system in man has been to differentiate between acute, short-lasting effects (which are usually a normal response) and chronic long-lasting alterations (which may be signs of cardiovascular pathology).

Experimental work in appropriate animal models has recently served to increase our knowledge in this respect. Most animals demonstrate a connection between the mid-brain and the cardiovascular system, especially during threats of different kinds. The so-called defence reaction constitutes a neurohormonal arousal as a preparation for flight or attack. The central vagal activity decreases at the same time as the sympathetic activity increases to the heart, venous capacitance vessels, kidney, intestines and skin, leading to decreased blood flow in these organs at the same time as the skeletal muscle blood flow increases. The difference between humans and animals, and especially in contemporary society, is that humans may suppress all outward signs of this reaction when they are threatened, even when the inner organism reacts in the same primitive way as do the animals. Behind a well-controlled poker face the ordinary individual still has tachycardia, increased blood pressure and alteration of the circulation and function of many vital organs.

To what extent these reactions really predispose to organic changes has so far mostly been a question of conjecture. New experimental data are, however, appearing. They demonstrate that, in certain circumstances, psychosocial influences may cause anatomical changes in the blood vessels and the heart. The American physiologist J.P. Henry [8] was one of the first to observe that monkeys trained for the space programme in the US developed arterial hypertension in several instances. Influenced by this observation, he developed specially designed social environments for colonies of mice, where he could manipulate the interrelationships between members of the group. He was able to demonstrate that strains of mice with usually low blood pressure developed progressive and irreversible hypertension when they were faced with increased social confrontations in a crowded surrounding where the animals had to compete for space, and for suitable mates. Other scientists have since used the experiences that Henry gained in these investigations. More detailed experiments have been conducted in order to get closer to the pathophysiological pathways that govern the cardiovascular disorders that may be initiated through these psychosocial mechanisms.

Kaplan et al. [9] have thus studied the influence of social stress in monkeys and demonstrated that the animals developed atherosclerotic manifestations in the aorta and the coronary arteries when they were subjected to a labile social environment through repeated changes in the relationship between individuals in the group of animals. They found that dominant, highly aggressive and competitive male monkeys had exacerbated coronary atherosclerosis, as measured by the cross-sectional intimal area, if they were maintained under conditions of social instability. Kaplan et al. equated this situation with a feeling of stress among the animals. There was also a clear difference between the dominant animals and the subordinates in the same group, indicating the importance of the personality of individual animals, which was probably expressed both in psychological and physiological terms.

In further experiments these authors have been able to show that an atherogenic diet may add to the changes seen [10]. Although such a diet may add to vascular pathology it did not in itself cause the arterial changes to develop. They have also demonstrated that at least some of these changes are mediated through the sympathetic nervous system, and can be reversed or prevented when the animals are treated with a $\beta$-adrenoceptor blocking substance. The influence of female hormones in female monkeys has also been studied, indicating a certain protective action of these hormones, at least under the circumstances of the study.

These investigations are time-consuming and complicated and the new information gained from them has to be critically evaluated in relation to our knowledge about the possible chain of events in humans: it has to be realized that no animal model exactly mimics the atherogenic process in humans. So far the results gained indicate that arousal of the sympathetic nervous system in man, such as occurs with intense behavioural stimulation or through different cardiovascular responses to psychosocial challenges, may be directly involved in the atherogenic process. Further studies are necessary to explore the extent to which these mechanisms are operating in man, their interrelation with other factors of importance, and whether and by what means they may be influenced. This might be possible in controlled investigations where human beings are monitored for the occurrence of coronary heart disease.

To sum up, our knowledge regarding background factors for atherosclerotic diseases in man is increasing rapidly. This is also the case for coronary heart disease and its clinical manifestations. It is now obvious that not only high blood pressure, elevated blood lipids and cigarette smoking are of importance for the premature development of coronary heart disease. The social environment, especially in the form of job strain that has been defined by Karasek and Theorell, the daily social network and, in animal experiments, environmental stress, can all play a powerful role in the development of arterial disease, probably and at least partly through arousal of the sympathetic nervous system. The physiological and psychological make-up of the individual, the social situation both at work and during leisure time, and the daily habits of the individual, good as well as bad, are all of importance both for the development of arterial lesions and for the occurrence of symptoms from the cardiovascular system (fig. 3).

More studies are needed both in animals and in man, to define more clearly the exact relationships between all these different factors in the initiation and development of atherosclerotic disease, and to analyse to what extent they might be influenced as part of a preventive programme. Until we know more about the details of these complex relationships between different mechanisms, it would be wise to keep a balanced view regarding the relative importance of the different factors for the development of symptoms in man. Exaggerated views either for or against any of

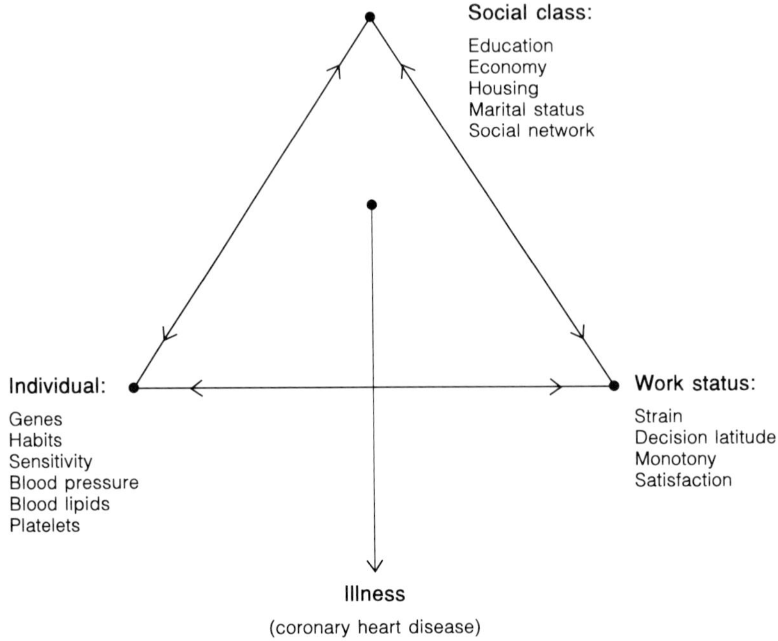


*Fig. 3.* Individual and environmental factors in development of coronary heart disease.

these contributing factors may do more harm than good in our attempts to understand the complicated origin of coronary heart disease in all its ramifications.

## *References*

1 Wilhelmsen L, Berglund G, Elmfeldt D, Tibblin G, Wedel H, Pennert K, Vedin A, Wilhelmsson C, Werko L: The multifactorial primary prevention trial in Göteborg, Sweden. Eur Heart J 1986;7:279–288.
2 Seyle H: The Stress of Life. New York, McGraw-Hill, 1936, republished 1976.
3 Karasek R, Theorell T: Healthy Work. New York, Basic Books Inc, 1990.
4 Karasek RA: Job demands, job decision latitude, and mental strain. Implications for job design. Adm Sci Q 1979;24:285–307.
5 Alfredsson L, Karasek R, Theorell T: Myocardial infarction risk and psychosocial work environment. Soc Sci Med 1982;16:463–467.
6 Karasek R, Theorell T, Schwartz JE, Schnall PL, Pieper CF, Michela JL: Job characteristics in relation to the prevalence of myocardial infarction in the US Health Examination Survey and the Health and Nutrition Examination Survey. Am J Public Health 1988;78:910–918.

7 Kristensen TS: Cardiovascular disease and the work environment. Scan J Work Environ Health 1989;15:165–179.
8 Henry JP, Ely DL, Stephens PM, Ratcliffe HL, Santisteban GA, Shapiro AP: The role of psychosocial factors in the development of arteriosclerosis in CBA mice. Atherosclerosis 1971;14:203–206.
9 Kaplan JR, Manuck SB, Clarkson TB, Lusso FM, Taub DM: Social status, environment and atherosclerosis in cynomolgus monkeys. Arteriosclerosis 1982;2:359–364.
10 Clarkson TB, Kaplan JR, Adams MR, Manuck SB: Psychosocial influences on the pathogenesis of atherosclerosis among nonhuman primates. Circulation 1987;76(suppl 1):29–40.

Prof. Lars Werko, The Swedish Council on Technology Assessment in Health Care, Box 16158, Hovslagar-gatan 2, S–10324 Stockholm (Sweden)

## *Discussion*

*Alberti* (Newcastle upon Tyne): Do you think that people who already demonstrate one of the other risk factors, such as hypertension, will be more affected by a stressful situation than those who do not?

*Werko* (Stockholm): It is important in all discussion of risk factors to distinguish between subjects who already have disease and ones who do not: for instance, the hypertensive patient with labile angina might react immediately to stress. These studies are aiming at individuals who have not yet developed any signs of disease, to see whether stressful situations may contribute to the development of, for instance, atheroma or arrhythmia.

*Roe* (London): Is this approach rather simplistic? In ordinary medical practice one sees that sources of stress often arise at home and concern the family or even travel to work: for some people, work is even a relief from stress at home.

*Werko:* I agree that one can have job strain at home, where one can't escape from pressure. I also agree that the model is simplistic, but so are almost all studies trying to analyse one factor alone because a conglomeration of factors is important.

*Bruckdorfer* (London): There were early studies looking at the relationship between stress and plasma catecholamine and free fatty acid levels, thinking that these might increase arrhythmias. Are there any recent measures of these plasma levels in relation to occupation?

*Werko:* Yes, but almost all studies have been during acute forms of stress so it is difficult to draw conclusions: for instance, it has been demonstrated in Stockholm bus drivers that catecholamine excretion increased with increased stress and increased incidence of coronary heart disease, so it is possible to find some link. Again, these studies could be regarded as simplistic, they are only looking at one hormone.

*Bruckdorfer:* There was a study of London bus drivers versus conductors: conductors came off better, perhaps because exercise burned off free fatty acids?

*Levy* (Birmingham): Looking at your figure 3, one is struck by the complexity of the situation in trying to alter work stress. Psychologists may have a rational approach in advising reorganization of work or stress reduction programmes, which can reduce blood pressure over time, showing that it is possible to alter one outcome measure.

Weetman DF, Wood D (eds): Risk Factors for Cardiovascular Disease in Non-Smokers. Int. Workshop, Washington, Tyne and Wear, 1991. Basel, Karger, 1993, pp 108–117

# Lead and Cardiovascular Disease

*Leonard S. Levy*

Institute of Occupational Health, University of Birmingham, UK

The possible role of lead as a causative factor in cardiovascular disease, and particularly in increased blood pressure, is both complex and controversial. The state of the current debate is best illustrated by reference to a 1990 leader in the *British Medical Journal* by Prof. W.R. Lee and Dr. M.R. Moore [1] and the subsequent letter of response by Dr. Dan Sharp [2]. Lee and Moore's leader essentially addressed the neurological research problems associated with low-level lead exposure. The article used Needleman's [3] 1979 work on cognitive functioning in children in relation to lead absorption as a starting point to consider current studies for and against the hypothesis that even low increases in lead uptake may be related to slight, but measurable, decrements in intellectual functioning. The article was detailed and thoughtful but made no mention of other possible effects of lead exposure. It was thus illuminating to read the letter of response from Dr. Sharp, who asserted that 'low-level lead exposure can result in hypertension' and who noted that this was not reported in the leader. He then stated: 'Europeans and North Americans have differing attitudes to the relation between lead and hypertension. Europeans tend to be uncritically dismissive and trivialise the relation, whereas North Americans uncritically embrace the association and consider that it has an appreciable impact on public health.'

Clearly, there appears to be a divergence of opinion regarding the effects of lead on the cardiovascular system and, in particular, its role as a possible contributor to hypertension. Thus, I will attempt to highlight the problem, particularly the 'North American view' as illustrated by the US Environmental Protection Agency (EPA) in their 'Air Quality Criteria for Lead' document of June 1986 [4], and supplemented with the 'Toxicology Profile for Lead' document, produced by the Agency for Toxic Substances and Disease Registry, 1988 [5]. I will then include additional information from the more recent literature.

Firstly, it would be useful to put these putative lower level effects into the context of the general toxicology of lead, a knowledge of which comes from occupationally-exposed groups of workers or experimental models.

## *Toxicology of Lead*

The harmful effects of lead, particularly following occupational exposures, have been well recognized for many years, and many countries have developed regulatory standards to deal with these harmful outcomes. More recently, environmental standards have been produced by bodies such as the EPA (in the US) and the CEC for the purposes of controlling emissions in the ambient air. The indisputable harmful effects can be classified as affecting the following target organs:

### *Blood*

Lead can inhibit haem synthesis by interference with sulphydryl groups in enzymes. At least five stages of haem synthesis are affected by lead but the two most sensitive enzymes are $\delta$-aminolaevulinic acid dehydratase and ferrochelatase. Such defective haem synthesis can lead to anaemia in lead poisoning but, in addition, synthesis of globin is also affected. The third way in which lead can cause anaemia, especially following heavy exposure, is to shorten the life-span of the red cell. It should be noted that anaemia is a late sign of lead intoxication.

### *Nervous System*

Lead can produce, in the peripheral nervous system, both axonal degeneration and segmental demyelination. Commonly, the motor nerves are affected and historically this led to 'wrist drop' in house painters who used lead-based paints. There is also evidence that lead can interfere with normal metabolism of some central neurotransmitters, including acetylcholine and catecholamines. The principal lesions in lead encephalopathy are cerebral oedema and perivascular haemorrhage, and areas of demyelination have been noted.

### *Kidney*

Lead has two principal effects on the kidney. Firstly, tubular damage involving mainly proximal cells and producing a Fanconi syndrome with aminoaciduria, glycosuria and phosphaturia. This syndrome has generally been seen in severely poisoned children. Secondly, it can cause a chronic interstitial nephropathy. This latter was once common in workers in

*Table 1.* Approximate blood lead levels and associated effects [after 6]

| Blood lead level | | Effect |
|---|---|---|
| μg/100 ml | μmol/l | |
| 10 | 0.5 | Elevation of zinc protoporphyrin |
| 20 | 1.0 | Inhibition of δ-aminolaevulinic acid dehydratase |
| 40 | 1.9 | Elevation of δ-aminolaevulinic acid and coproporphyrin in the urine |
| 50 | 2.4 | Peripheral neuropathy (subclinical) |
| 60 | 2.9 | Shortening of red cell life-span |
| 80 | 3.9 | Anaemia |
| 130 | 6.3 | Impairment of renal function |
| 150 | 7.2 | Encephalopathy |

uncontrolled lead industries. More serious cases led to renal failure or hypertensive disease.

### *Blood Lead Levels and Effects*

Although it is difficult to give exact figures, table 1 gives approximate figures within the dose-effect range for increasing severity of toxic effects from lead.

### *Lead Poisoning*

Classical inorganic lead poisonings, with abdominal symptoms including colic, nausea and vomiting, are now rare, as are the severe neurological symptoms such as wrist drop. However, slowing of nerve conduction velocity may be seen in occupationally-exposed groups who are symptomless. Based on his work in the mid-1970s, Waldron [6] has suggested that the threshold for the more proven subtle neurobehavioural effects is at around 40 μg/100 ml, although others have subsequently claimed subtle neurobehavioural changes at much lower levels, and Bell [7] has suggested a 'no effect level' in the range of 10–15 μg/100 ml in the blood in children – a level which may be found in many urban populations and related to environmental, not occupational, exposure. Environmental sources of lead in such circumstances are food, water and the air (related to petrol additives).

## *Cardiotoxicity and Lead*

### *Mortality Studies*

Lead has long been reported to have cardiovascular effects at high exposure levels in industry: however, as the effects were mainly associated with lead-induced renal disease, it is difficult to evaluate independently the effect of lead per se on the cardiovascular system. In 1963, Dingwall-Fordyce and Lane [8] reported an increase in cerebrovascular disease in heavily exposed lead workers, but these workers received their exposure in the first quarter of the 20th century when occupational conditions were clearly much worse. In 1986, the EPA [4] noted that: 'There has been no similar increase in the mortality rate reported for men employed in recent times'. However, two more recent publications report on the mortality of workers with significant lead exposure. In the first of these, Cooper et al. [9] report on the mortality experience of two groups of lead-exposed workers between 1947 and 1980, a 34-year period. The study involved a cohort of 4,519 battery plant workers and 2,300 lead production workers. There were 1,718 deaths in the first cohort and 621 in the second. Mortality from all causes combined was significantly greater than expected in each cohort, with standardized mortality rates (SMRs) of 107 and 113 respectively. Among battery plant workers, the increase in mortality rate was mainly due to excess deaths from malignant neoplasms (SMR = 113) and hypertensive disease, mainly renal in origin (SMR = 320). Among the lead production workers, the pattern was similar but with a non-significant increase in neoplasms. In neither cohort was there a significant increase in cerebrovascular disease. Furthermore, a proportionate mortality analysis showed that excess deaths from cerebrovascular disease and from hypertensive heart disease among smelters were in part due to the high proportion of non-whites in the smelter populations. The authors concluded that ethnicity, diet, alcohol and cigarette smoking could not be ruled out as possible confounding aetiological factors for the cancer deaths.

In the other investigation, on the mortality of Swedish smelter workers, Gerhardsson et al. [10] selected a cohort of 437 heavily exposed lead workers who were employed between 1950 and 1974. They were divided into groups on the basis of cumulative blood lead doses, and SMRs were calculated. In the lead cohort, only the raised SMR for lung cancer was sustained (SMR = 162, not significant), but no significant differences were found between high-lead- and low-lead-exposed groups. Mean annual blood lead concentration for all lead workers was around 58.2 $\mu$g/100 ml blood in 1950, falling to 33.6 $\mu$g/100 ml blood in 1974. Of particular interest was the finding that for the lead-exposed workers, the SMRs for circulatory disease, ischaemic heart disease and cerebrovascular disease was less than 100. Thus, whatever other effects lead exposure, occupational or environmental, may have on the cardiovascular system, the studies cited do not indicate an obvious direct cardiovascular mortality for occupationally-exposed groups.

*Other Cardiovascular Effects*

There have been reports of both structural and functional cardiovascular changes in adults and children with acute lead poisoning. Myocardial abnormalities have been noted in cases of clinical lead poisoning and, because ECG abnormalities have disappeared on chelation therapy, an aetiological relationship with lead is strengthened. Kline [11] reported degenerative changes in heart muscle in 5 fatal cases of lead poisoning in children. It is unclear whether such changes are a specific response to lead even though electron microscopy on lead-intoxicated mice has shown diffuse degenerative changes in the myocardium [12]. In further support of a direct myocardial effect, Kosmider and Petelenz [13] have reported that 66% of a group of adults aged 46 and over with pre-existing lead poisoning of occupational origin had ECG abnormalities – a rate that was four times the age-adjusted rate. More recently, a study [14] of 95 lead smelters (with a mean blood lead level of 51 μg/100 ml) and a group of matched unexposed controls (with a mean blood lead level of 11 μg/100 ml) showed a significantly higher incidence of ischaemic ECG changes (20% exposed vs. 6% unexposed). It is also worth noting that in addition to ECG changes, a slight (4–5 mm Hg) but significant increase in diastolic pressure was recorded in the lead-exposed group compared to the controls. Systolic blood pressure showed no such changes.

In a further occupational investigation of lead- and cadmium-exposed workers [15], 53 lead- and cadmium-exposed male workers from a lead processing plant (with a mean blood level of 47.4 μg/100 ml) were compared to 52 non-lead-exposed workers (mean blood level 8.1 μg/100 ml). Blood pressure levels were positively correlated with blood lead and urinary cadmium levels.

A prospective study by Weiss et al. [16] of 89 Boston policemen demonstrated that high blood lead level ( $>30$ μg/100 ml) was a significant predictor of subsequent elevation in systolic blood pressure. Low blood lead level (20–29 μg/100 ml) was not. There was no effect on diastolic blood pressure, a finding that is at variance with that of Kirby and Gyntelberg [14]. The authors tested for both smoking and alcohol consumption and, on balance, felt that the lead was the aetiological factor. They considered possible physiological mechanisms which they stated were unknown, but suggested that the effect was unlikely to be related to renal function (not measured) in their healthy working population of men. They favoured the possibility of a number of direct effects of lead on blood pressure and cited as supporting evidence: (a) increases in systolic pressure in rats, associated with low plasma renin levels, but without renal damage [17]; (b) increased vascular responsiveness in rats, suggestive of abnormal sympathetic nervous system activity [18]; (c) increased levels of catecholamines and decreased baroreceptor responsiveness in subjects with increased blood lead levels [19], and (d) low plasma renin and aldosterone levels in lead-exposed individuals [20].

More recent work on occupationally-exposed lead workers raises the possibility that lead could affect blood pressure via the renin-angiotensin system, as shown by lead-related increases in plasma renin and angiotensin I levels [21], and the kallikrein-kinin system, as demonstrated by a correlation between renin and kallikrein [22]. Further evidence for an association between lead and systolic blood pressure comes from investigations by Moreau et al. [23] and Orssaud et al. [24] on 431 male civil servant employees of the Paris Police Department. There was an increase in blood pressure from the first blood lead group ($<12.4\ \mu g/100$ ml) to the fourth ($24.8-30.8\ \mu g/100$ ml), with an overall increase in systolic blood pressure of 9 mm Hg.

There have been two major general population studies: in the UK, the British Regional Heart Study [25, 26] and in the US, The National Health and Nutrition Examination Survey II (NHANES II). This latter study has been analysed in a variety of ways [27–30]. A simple correlation analysis of the NHANES II data by Harlan et al. [27] demonstrated a significant linear association between blood lead levels and both systolic and diastolic blood pressure levels for men and women aged 12–74 years. After multiple regression analysis to allow for some confounding factors, significant association remained only for men. Analysis of the NHANES II data set by Pirkle et al. [28] set out to examine the relationship between blood lead levels and blood pressure in white males aged 40–59 years (564 men). Multiple regression analysis showed significant correlation between blood lead and blood pressure and, further, no threshold was demonstrated below which lead level was not significantly related to systolic or diastolic blood pressure. Disturbingly, the analysis also suggested that large initial increments in blood pressure occurred at relatively modest blood lead levels. Lead was considered a significant predictor of diastolic blood pressure greater than 90 mm Hg.

Pirkle et al. [28] further produced a predicted number of fatal and nonfatal myocardial infarctions for a 10-year follow-up period and mean blood lead levels for this population. Based on this, the EPA [4] concluded that white males, aged 40–59, were at increased risk in that these blood pressure elevations were significantly correlated with elevations in blood lead levels.

The UK study involved 7,735 men, aged 40–59, from 24 British towns. Blood lead levels were obtained for 7,371 men. The EPA [4] reported that this study demonstrated a small but significant correlation between systolic blood pressure and blood lead levels and of the 74 men with blood lead levels greater than 37 $\mu$g/100 ml, a higher proportion had systolic or diastolic hypertension than did all other men combined. It is, however, worth noting Pocock's [26] own early observations on his data: 'The association is very weak, the study is observational and it is difficult to adjust for all relevant confounders. Therefore, it is premature to conclude that an elevated body lead burden has a causal influence on blood pressure.'

Interestingly, the EPA [4] were more cautious in proposing a mechanism, based on the human and animal toxicology, by which lead caused hypertension. This was summarized by ATSDR [5] as: '. . . although lead, even at very low levels, produces effects on the renin-angiotensin system in animals, these changes are not established as the cause of hypertension. Rather, hypertension is more likely to be due to changes in vascular reactivity and level of sympathetic tone, both of which may be dependent on lead-related changes in intracellular calcium ion concentration.'

Since these reviews were completed, further evidence has emerged. In a study of some 1,721 male and female subjects in Wales [31], there was no association between blood pressure and blood lead levels. Within this study, there was a cohort of 1,104 men (from the Caerphilly Collaborative Heart Disease Study) aged 49–63. Again, there was no association between blood level and either resting blood pressure or the rise in blood pressure during a cold pressor test.

A further general population study has been reported by Grandjean et al. [32], based on 1,052 men and women born in 1936 and residing in the Glostrup area of Denmark. All were examined in 1976 at age 40 and then 966 were re-examined 5 years later. Examination included blood lead assessment and blood pressure measurements. Complete blood pressure and blood lead levels were available for 861 subjects (451 men and 410 women). Median blood levels were 13 and 9 $\mu$g/100 ml at age 40 years and 9 and 6 $\mu$g/100 ml at age 45 years for men and women respectively. The drop in blood lead in both men and women coincided with the reduction in the amount of lead additives used in petrol. The results showed that there was a slightly increased blood lead concentration in women with a systolic blood pressure above 140 mm Hg and/or a diastolic blood pressure above 90 mm Hg. Systolic blood pressure in men and women and diastolic blood pressure in women correlated significantly with log [blood lead] at age 40 years but not at age 45 years, a doubling in blood lead being associated with an increase in blood pressure of 3 mm Hg or less. However,

Grandjean pointed out that, of nine potential confounding factors assessed, only blood haemoglobin and alleged alcohol intake were significantly associated with both blood lead levels and blood pressure. If either or both of these confounding factors were entered into a multiple regression analysis, then the blood lead/blood pressure association became non-significant. He thus concluded that as both haemoglobin levels and alcohol intake appeared to be biologically plausible confounders, 'any independent effect of low-level lead exposure on blood pressure could not be determined'. He produced cogent arguments for his views and contended that 'the available evidence supports the notion that at least high alcohol intake is an independent cause of increased blood pressure *and also* of increased blood lead levels' and 'Almost all lead in the blood is bound to the erythrocytes, and misleadingly low blood (lead) levels may be seen in anaemia; adjustment of blood lead to a certain haemoglobin level is therefore appropriate'. However, he did not rule out the possibility of a causal role of low levels of lead exposure with regard to a small increase in blood pressure, but he certainly urged caution in accepting a direct causal relationship without further investigation.

In conclusion, the issue is clearly a complex one. Attempting to tease out the effect of just one component from the multiple causal factors contributing to elevated blood pressure is extremely difficult: the more so, the lower the elevation in blood lead level considered. However, the conclusions that can reasonably be drawn from the available data are: (1) On balance, there do appear to be small, but measurable, increases in systolic and diastolic blood pressures with increasing blood lead concentrations. (2) The exposure level at which these occur can be described as low, and certainly in the 'subclinical' range. (3) There are a number of important confounding factors which could all contribute to both an increase in blood lead and an increase in blood pressure – thus the association may be concomitant rather than causal. (4) There is experimental evidence which suggests several biological mechanisms by which blood lead increases could induce blood pressure increases, either alone or with other factors.

Certainly, the public health implications warrant further investigation to clarify this complex issue.

## *References*


1 Lee WR, Moore MR: Low level exposure to lead. The evidence for harm accumulates (Leader). BMJ 1990;301:504–506.

2 Sharp DS: Low level exposure to lead (letter). BMJ 1990;301:985.

3 Needleman HJ, Gunnue C, Levitan A, Reed R, Peresie H, Maher C, Barrett BS: Deficits in psychologic and classroom performance of children with elevated dentive lead levels. N Engl J Med 1979;300:689–695.

4 EPA: Air Quality Criteria for Lead. United States Environmental Protection Agency. Environmental Criteria and Assessment Office. 1986.
5 ATSDR: Toxicological Profile for Lead. Agency for Toxic Substances and Disease Registry. United States Public Health Service, Oak Ridge National Laboratory, 1988.
6 Waldron HA: Lead; in Waldron HA (ed): Metals in the Environment. London, Academic Press, 1980, pp 155–197.
7 Bell A: Toxicity of lead at low dose. Br J Ind Med 1990;47:288.
8 Dingwall-Fordyce I, Lane RE: A follow-up study of lead workers. Br J Ind Med 1963;20:313–315.
9 Cooper WC, Wong O, Kheifets L: Mortality among employees of lead battery plants and lead-producing plants, 1947–1980. Scand J Work Environ Health 1985;11:331–345.
10 Gerhardsson L, Lundstrom N-G, Norberg G, Wall S: Mortality and lead exposure: A retrospective cohort study of Swedish smelter workers. Br J Ind Med 1986;43:707–712.
11 Kline TS: Myocardial changes in lead poisoning. Am J Dis Child 1960;99:48–54.
12 Khan MY, Buse M, Louria DB: Lead cardiomyopathy in mice. Arch Pathol Lab Med 1977;101:89–94.
13 Kosmider S, Petelenz T: Electrocardiographic changes in elderly patients with chronic professional lead poisoning. Pol Arch Med Wewn 1962;32:437–442.
14 Kirkby H, Gyntelberg F: Blood pressure and other cardiovascular risk factors of long-term exposure to lead. Scand J Work Environ Health 1985;11:15–19.
15 de Kort WLAM, Verschoor MA, Wibowo AAE, van Hemmen JJ: Occupational exposure to lead and blood pressure. A study of 105 workers. Am J Ind Med 1987;11:145–156.
16 Weiss ST, Munoz A, Stein A, Sparrow D, Speizer FE: The relationship of blood lead to blood pressure in a longitudinal study of working men. Am J Epidemiol 1986;123:800–808.
17 Victery W, Vander AJ, Markel LK, Shulak JM, Germain C: Lead exposure, begun in utero, decreases renin and angiotensin II in adult rats. Proc Soc Exp Biol Med 1982;170:63–67.
18 Webb RC, Winquist RJ, Victery W, Vander AJ: In vivo and in vitro effects of lead on vascular reactivity in rats. Am J Physiol 1981;241:H211–H216.
19 Bertel O, Buhler FR, Ott JC: Lead-induced hypertension: Blunted beta-adrenoreceptor-mediated functions. BMJ 1978;i:551.
20 Sandstead HH, Michelakis AM, Temple TG: Lead intoxication: Its effects on the renin-aldosterone response and sodium deprivation. Arch Environ Health 1970;20:356–363.
21 Campbell BC, Meredith PA, Scott JJC: Lead exposure and changes in the renin-angiotensin-aldosterone system in man. Toxicol Lett 1985;25:25–32.
22 Boscolo P, Galli G, Iannaccone A, Martino, F, Porcelli F, Trancore L: Plasma renin activity and urinary kallikrein excretion in lead-exposed workers as related to hypertension and nephropathy. Life Sci 1981;28:175–184.
23 Moreau T, Orssaud G, Juguet B, Busquet G: Blood lead levels and arterial pressure: Initial results of a cross-sectional study of 431 male subjects. Rev Epidemiol Sante Publique 1982;39:395–397.
24 Orssaud G, Claude JR, Moreau T, Tellouch J, Juguet B, Festy B: Blood lead concentrations and blood pressure. BMJ 1985;290:244.
25 Pocock SJ, Shaper AG, Ashby D, Delves T, Whitehead TP: Blood lead concentration, blood pressure and renal function. BMJ 1984;289:872–874.
26 Pocock SJ, Shaper AG, Ashby D, Delves T: Blood lead and blood pressure in middle-aged men; in Lekkas TD (ed): International Conference on Heavy Metals in the Environment, Athens, Greece. Edinburgh, CEP Consultants Ltd, 1985, vol 1, pp 303–305.

27 Harlan WR, Landis JR, Schmouder RL, Goldsten NG, Harlan LC: Blood lead and blood pressure: Relationship in the adolescent and adult US population. J Am Med Assoc 1985;23S:530–534.

28 Pirkle JL, Schwartz J, Landis JR, Harlan WR: The relationship between blood lead levels and blood pressure and its cardiovascular risk implications. Am J Epidemiol 1985;121:246–258.

29 Landis JR, Flegal KM: A generalised Mantel-Haenszel analysis of the regression of blood pressure on blood lead using NHANES II data. Environ Health Perspect 1988;78:35–41.

30 Schwartz J: Blood lead and blood pressure in middle-aged men; in Lekkas TD (ed): International Conference on Heavy Metals in the Environment, Athens, Greece. Edinburgh, CEP Consultants Ltd, 1985, vol 1, pp 300–302.

31 Elwood PC, Yarnell JWG, Oldham PD, Catford JC, Nutbeam D, Davey-Smith G, Toothill C: Blood pressure and blood lead in surveys in Wales. Am J Epidemiol 1988;127:942–945.

32 Grandjean P, Hollnagel H, Hedgegaard L, Christensen JM, Larsen S: Lead-blood pressure relations: Alcohol intake and hemoglobin as confounders. Am J Epidemiol 1989;129:732–739.

Dr. Leonard S. Levy, Institute of Occupational Health,
University of Birmingham, Birmingham B15 2TT (UK)

Weetman DF, Wood D (eds): Risk Factors for Cardiovascular Disease in Non-Smokers. Int. Workshop, Washington, Tyne and Wear, 1991. Basel, Karger, 1993, pp 118–128

# Carbon Monoxide Exposure as a Risk Factor for Cardiovascular Disease

*F.J.C. Roe*

Consultant in Toxicology, Wimbledon Common, London, UK

In this paper I shall attempt to answer the following questions: (1) What are the short-term effects of carbon monoxide (CO) and how long does it stay in the body? (2) Are the short-term effects of exposure to low ambient levels of CO harmful to normal individuals or to individuals with reduced cardiovascular function? (3) Does repeated exposure to CO predispose to atherosclerosis and/or myocardial infarction in humans or animals? (4) How and to what extent are non-smokers exposed to CO from other people's tobacco smoke, other indoor sources or vehicular exhaust fumes?

## *What Are the Short-Term Effects of CO and How Long Does It Stay in the Body?*

Oxygen ($O_2$) is transported from the lungs to the tissues in the form of a relatively loose association with haemoglobin (Hb). The $O_2$ diffuses through the normally thin alveolar wall into the serum, and from there it is taken up by the Hb in the red blood corpuscles. The amount of $O_2$ taken up by each gram of Hb is determined by the concentration of $O_2$ in the serum which, in turn, is determined by its concentration in the alveoli. The amount of $O_2$ carried to other tissues is determined by the amount taken up by each gram of Hb, by the amount of Hb per unit volume of blood, and by the rate of blood flow. Removal of $O_2$ from oxygenated Hb is influenced by the $O_2$ tension in the tissues through which it passes. Heavy use of $O_2$ results in reduced $O_2$ tension and increased dissociation of oxygenated Hb as blood passes through the tissue concerned. The heart is a heavy user of $O_2$.

Unfortunately, Hb has an affinity for CO (to form carboxyhaemoglobin (COHb)) that is over 200 times its affinity for $O_2$. Thus, COHb is readily formed even under conditions where the tension of CO in the alveoli is relatively low. Hb that has combined with CO is not available for carrying $O_2$. Apart from the effects of the replacement of oxyhaemoglobin by COHb, there is evidence that the presence of CO in the blood slows the release of $O_2$ from oxyhaemoglobin. CO also combines reversibly with myoglobin, a protein in muscle cells. It has been suggested that this effect per se contributes to the toxic effects of CO on, for instance, the functioning of the heart [1]. COHb eventually dissociates again into CO and Hb on prolonged exposure to air which is substantially free from CO. In other words, CO is gradually lost by the same route as it is acquired.

The rate of loss of CO (i.e. the rate of dissociation of COHb) is dependent not only on the difference between the concentrations of CO in both the blood and the alveolar air, but also on the rates of respiration and blood flow through the lungs. Exercise, by increasing the respiration rate, hastens the loss of CO; lack of exercise retards it. During deep sleep, even in a CO-free atmosphere, COHb levels fall only very slowly. According to Dr P.V. Cole [pers. commun.], COHb levels fall faster in men than women, presumably because the number of red blood cells per unit volume of blood is lower in women.

CO combines even more avidly with fetal Hb than with adult Hb. Cole et al [2] found COHb levels in the fetus to be 80% higher than those in the mother after a pregnant woman has been exposed to CO. Also, after exposure ceases, the COHb concentration falls more slowly in the fetus than in the mother.

The anatomy of the lungs is ideal for gaseous exchange between the blood and the atmosphere (i.e. alveolar air): $O_2$ passes readily in and carbon dioxide ($CO_2$) passes readily out. CO enjoys the same easy passage in both directions, but the strength of its association with Hb severely limits the rate it is lost from the body.

According to Dalhamn et al [3], absorption of CO through the epithelium of the nose and pharynx is negligible: it is also negligible in the trachea and bronchi down as far as the respiratory bronchioles, although there is no information available on this [G. Cumming, pers. commun.]. It is reasonable to assume that little CO would escape from the body except via the lungs. Less than 0.1% of absorbed CO is oxidized to $CO_2$.

Apart from the CO which is taken into the body from the surrounding air, it is noteworthy that some CO is formed endogenously as a by-product of haem metabolism [4, 5].

### *Are the Short-Term Effects of Exposure to Low Ambient Levels of CO Harmful to Normal Individuals or to Individuals with Compromised Cardiovascular Function?*

*In Normal Individuals*

The normal body is able to compensate for changes in oxygen demand and supply by increasing the respiration rate (to raise alveolar $O_2$ tension), by increasing blood flow (by increasing heart rate and stroke volume) and, over a longer period, by increasing numbers of red blood cells and Hb per unit volume of blood. These compensatory changes are very similar to the adaptive changes which occur when people living at low altitudes climb to higher altitudes where the air is more rarified. The changes are reversible and there is no evidence, or real likelihood, that permanent or accumulative effects are produced in healthy individuals, provided that peak COHb levels do not rise above 10%. It is only in some heavy smokers that COHb levels regularly reach as high as this, and, although heavy smoking is associated with increased incidence of coronary heart disease, cerebrovascular disease and peripheral vascular disease, it is not known whether this association is with exposure to CO or with that to other components of tobacco smoke.

Ayres et al. [6] reported that a rise of COHb concentration to 9% is associated with an increase in coronary blood flow in humans, while Adams et al. [7] showed that a 5% increase in COHb was associated with a 14% increase in coronary blood flow in dogs.

Although it has not been proven that intermittent low peak levels of COHb do no permanent harm, it seems likely that the healthy body can compensate for them completely.

Cohen et al. [8] found an increased fatality rate from myocardial infarction in areas with high rates of air pollution, but only during periods of high CO pollution. However, they were uncertain whether the association indicated a cause-effect relationship.

*In Individuals with Compromised Cardiovascular Function*

Theoretically one would anticipate that in subjects with atherosclerotic coronary vessels which are unable to expand or contract, there could be no compensatory increase in coronary blood flow as COHb levels rise. In turn, this could lead to a reduction in the functional cardiac reserve and an earlier onset of anginal pain upon exercising. In line with this expectation, Ayres et al. [9] reported disturbed lactate and pyruvate metabolism, indicative of myocardial hypoxia, when COHb levels rose in subjects known to have coronary heart disease. Also, Anderson et al. [10] and Allred et al. [11] saw ECG changes (increased S-T depression) in anginal patients when they were exposed to 50 ppm CO in ambient air. Calverley et al. [12] observed reduced exercise tolerance in 15 patients with severe chronic bronchitis and emphysema after they had been exposed to enough CO to raise their COHb levels to 9%. Allred et al. [11] found that a rise in the COHb level to between 2 and 3%, as could occur in subjects confined to heavily contaminated air in a badly ventilated room, was enough to reduce exercise tolerance.

A difficulty with the interpretation of laboratory studies of the kind that have been reported by Ayres et al. [9], Anderson et al. [10] and Aronow [13] is that simply being in an investigative laboratory is stressful for subjects with compromised cardiovascular function. The release of catecholamines as a result of this stress and the consequential increase in blood pressure is apt to complicate the interpretation of the findings in such studies. The same problem virtually prevents any meaningful investigation of the possible effects of CO derived from other people's tobacco smoke on cardiovascular parameters in either normal subjects or patients with existing cardiovascular disease. The characteristic smell of tobacco serves to inform the subject when he/she is being exposed to CO as distinct from uncontaminated air, and if he/she has been conditioned to believe that environmental tobacco smoke is dangerous, fear or annoyance caused by the smell of it may trigger off a rise in blood pressure.

### *Does Repeated Exposure to CO Predispose to Atherosclerosis and/or Myocardial Infarction?*

#### *In Humans*

Autopsy studies suggest that there is an association between cigarette smoking and increased atherosclerosis of the aorta and coronary arteries. However, this does not tell us whether CO, per se, is implicated in the causation of atherosclerosis and at least one other component of tobacco smoke, namely nicotine, attracts as much attention as CO in this context.

Theoretically, raised COHb could predispose to atherosclerosis in various ways: (a) By reducing oxygen tension and thereby damaging the lining of arteries or the deeper structures of the walls of arteries. (b) By an effect on circulating blood lipids. (c) By increasing the risk of mural thrombus formation either by increasing platelet stickiness or by some other mechanism.

Evidence that exposure of humans to CO predisposes to atherosclerosis has been provided by a study reported by Wald et al. [14]. In this study, 1,085 subjects were questioned about their smoking habits and history of symptoms of vascular disease. They were then physically examined and asked to provide a sample of venous blood. A better correlation was found between COHb concentration in the blood and evidence of atherosclerotic disease than between smoking history and such disease. As the authors of this paper themselves point out, their findings do not prove that CO per se is atherogenic. COHb levels are not only an index of the inhalation of the CO in tobacco smoke, they are also an index of absorption of nicotine from the smoke. The evidence of Wald et al [14], therefore, does not point more strongly at CO than at nicotine, or any other component of cigarette smoke, for that matter.

The mechanisms involved in the development of atherosclerosis are the subject of continuing debate. According to several theories, high levels of circulating cholesterol and/or free fatty acids (FFA) predispose to atherosclerosis. A demonstration that CO, independently of dietary cholesterol intake, raises blood cholesterol and FFA levels could, according to these theories, be taken as evidence that exposure to CO predisposes to the development of atherosclerosis.

Kjeldsen and Damgaard [15] saw no significant changes in total fatty acids, phospholipids or triglycerides in the blood of 8 volunteers given 5 half-hour exposures to 0.5% CO on 8–10 successive days (COHb = 12.5%). However, there was a significant increase in serum cholesterol during the last 3 days of exposure.

*In Animals*

*Lipid Deposition in Walls of Arteries.* The results of some animal studies suggest that exposure to CO increases the risk of deposition of lipid in the walls of the aorta and coronary arteries when animals are fed a high-cholesterol diet. Cholesterol-fed rabbits continuously exposed to CO for 10 or 12 weeks [16, 17] and cholesterol-fed squirrel monkeys intermittently exposed to CO for 7 months [18] showed excessive deposition of lipid in the intima of the aorta and coronary arteries when compared with animals exposed to CO but fed on a normal diet, or with animals fed on a high-cholesterol diet without CO exposure. Malinow et al. [19] saw no evidence of atherosclerosis or raised serum cholesterol levels in cynomolgus monkeys when fed either a standard or a high-cholesterol diet and exposed to CO. Armitage et al. [20] observed more lipid in the intima of the aorta and coronary arteries of White Carneau pigeons fed a high-cholesterol diet than in control birds. Birds exposed for 52 weeks to both a high-cholesterol diet and CO showed marginally, but not significantly, more lipid deposition than birds exposed to cholesterol only. Exposure of birds on a normal diet to CO (COHb = 11–12%) had no effect on the arteries.

Webster et al. [18] exposed cholesterol-fed monkeys to CO over a 7-month period. They saw significantly more atherosclerosis of the coronary arteries in them than in cholesterol-fed monkeys exposed only to room air.

Kjeldsen et al. [15] reported that hypoxia, achieved without exposure to CO, also gave rise to increased lipid formation in the lining of the aorta in cholesterol-fed rabbits. Later, Kjeldson et al. [21] reported that hyperoxia (achieved by exposing animals to 28% $O_2$) protected cholesterol-fed rabbits against the development of lipid deposits in the wall of the aorta.

*Intimal Oedema.* Kjeldsen et al. [22] and later Hugod et al. [23], using the electron microscope, reported the occurrence of intimal oedema of the aorta in rabbits fed on a normal diet and exposed to 180 ppm CO continuously for 2 weeks. Later, however, Astrup and Kjeldsen [24] reported that they were unable to confirm that CO produces any effects on the intima of arteries.

Pfrender [25], in a critical résumé of chronic carbon monoxide poisoning, stated, 'Almost all pathologic lesions can be explained on the basis of simple tissue anoxia, as can the late sequelae'.

*Raised Haematocrit.* Other studies, such as those of Eckardt et al. [26] in which monkeys were exposed to CO for 2 years and those of Jones et al. [27] in which rats, guinea pigs, monkeys and dogs were exposed to CO for 90 days, have shown mainly negative results except for an elevation of mean Hb levels and haematocrit values. However, these are of no real value in relation to atherosclerosis, since no special attempt was made to assess the animals for the extent of lipid deposition in the aorta or coronary arteries at post-mortem, and information on the cholesterol content of the diets given to the animals was not provided.

*Serum Cholesterol.* According to Kjeldsen [28], continuous exposure of rabbits to CO may increase serum cholesterol concentrations either when the animals are given a normal diet or when they are given a diet containing 2% added cholesterol.

Since these various animal studies were conducted, the focus has moved away from cholesterol per se as the particular lipid likely to be implicated in atherosclerosis. Instead, suspicion falls far more heavily on low-density lipoproteins (LDLs). Unfortunately, no data have been reported from studies in which animals have been exposed to high LDL diets and CO.

*Platelets.* Birnstingl et al. [29] reported that after exposure to 400 ppm CO for 6–14 h, which increased their average COHb levels to 17.5%, rabbits showed a highly significant increase in platelet stickiness. This was followed 24 h later by a fall to significantly below the pre-exposure level. Immediately after exposure, platelet counts were normal, but 24 h later they were reduced to 60% of normal. This reduction is consistent with the possibility that hyper-sticky platelets had stuck to the walls of damaged blood vessels.

Kjeldsen et al. [22] saw platelets and red blood cells adhering to the lining of the aorta denuded of intima as a result of an exposure of animals (rabbits) to CO.

### *How and to What Extent Are Non-Smokers Exposed to CO from Other People's Tobacco Smoke, Other Indoor Sources or Vehicular Exhaust Fumes?*

#### *CO from Other People's Tobacco Smoke*

Various workers have measured CO levels in tobacco smoke-filled rooms and the COHb levels in non-smokers confined to such rooms. COHb levels of the same order as those of policemen on point duty (traffic direction) have generally been found.

Russell et al. [30], for instance, exposed 11 non-smokers for an average of 79 min to a smoky atmosphere 'made worse than would be likely encountered in natural social conditions' by closing all the windows and switching off the ventilation. The level of CO averaged 38 ppm. The mean initial COHb level in the 11 subjects was 1.6 (+0.6)% and this rose to a mean of 2.6 (+0.7)% after an average of 79 min. Srch [31] found 90 ppm CO in a stationary tobacco smoke-filled car with all the windows closed and a rise of from 2 to 5% in the COHb levels of 2 non-smoking occupants of the car during a period of 1 h. During the experiment, the car was kept with the engine turned off in a closed garage. The car was apparently a small one (internal volume = 2.09 $m^3$). Harke [32] reported a rise in the mean COHb concentration, from 0.9 to 2.1%, in 7 non-smokers housed for 90 min in a smoke-filled room. The concentration of CO averaged 30 ppm. Based on measurements of COHb and of nicotine (and presumably cotinine) in urine, Harke, in Dontenwill's laboratory, concluded that, in normally ventilated rooms, non-smokers absorb of the order of less than 1% of the amounts of smoke constituents absorbed by smokers. Because some components of smoke, and especially of side-stream smoke, e.g. acrolein, are irritants to the eyes and to the mucous membranes of the upper respiratory tract, persons confined to smoke-filled spaces tend to open windows. For this reason in particular, the extreme conditions of high smoke and CO concentrations used by some investigators are unrealistic.

*CO from Other Indoor Sources*

In the UK prior to the replacement of coal gas by natural gas, there were between 1,500 and 2,000 deaths from CO poisoning each year. By 1979, the number of deaths in England and Wales had fallen to about 100 [33].

Gas fires, kerosene heaters and open coal or wood fires are sources of CO, particularly under conditions of incomplete combustion. However, ambient levels only rise to potentially dangerous levels if chimneys and/or other ventilation outlets are blocked. In some oriental countries, such as Korea, heating is commonly achieved with the 'Ondol' system in which coal briquettes are burnt directly under the floor on which people sleep. The system is very economical but there is always a danger that CO will seep through unrecognised cracks in the floor. Many thousands of cases of CO poisoning caused in this way are admitted to hospitals in Korea and hundreds of people so affected die. In many regions of the world where ambient temperatures are very low during part or all of the year or where they can fall to low levels during the night, it is not uncommon for kitchens to be completely unventilated. Women who spend, sometimes, several hours in such kitchens are exposed to dangerous levels of fumes including, inter alia, high levels of CO.

*Vehicular Exhaust Fumes*

In western countries it is not uncommon for people to commit suicide by driving a car into a garage, closing and sealing the doors and then running the car engine in the enclosed space. Death from CO poisoning is easily achieved in this way.

In many big cities, especially in the Orient, there can be high ambient levels of CO in cars stuck in traffic jams in road tunnels and on the streets in general, and the latter can result in similarly high levels in the houses and shops lining streets with heavy traffic.

Levels of 25–100 ppm CO have been commonly found in London street air by Lawther and Commins [34] and in Toronto street air by Godin et al. [35]. Non-smoking policemen on point duty in heavy traffic conditions in London had COHb levels mainly between 1 and 2%, but one had 3.8% COHb [34]. Other studies have given similar results [36–39]. For instance, levels of up to 3% COHb are common in non-smokers exposed to vehicular exhaust gases in Los Angeles [40, 41].

## *Conclusion*

There is no clear evidence that exposure to CO is associated with an increased incidence of any form of cardiovascular disease. In the laboratory, the incidence of atheromatous-like deposits in the intima of arteries has been reported when animals have been exposed both to a high-cholesterol diet and to CO, but not where there is exposure only to CO. It is not certain, however, that the lesions produced by such double exposures are really analogous to any form of cardiovascular disease that occurs in humans.

At the present time, there is increasing interest in the possibility that lipid peroxidation is implicated in the aetiology both of ageing-related diseases, such as atherosclerosis and cancer. The oxidants involved can be either exogenous or endogenous in origin. In either case, protection is afforded by antioxidants and particularly by vitamin E. CO is neither an oxidant nor an antioxidant. Hence, if the above theory is right, there is no a priori reason to expect CO to influence the risk of atherosclerosis in either direction.

## *References*


1 Susuki T: Effects of carbon monoxide inhalation on the fine structure of the rat heart muscle. Tohoku J Exp Med 1969;97:197–211.

2 Cole PV, Hawkins LH, Roberts D: Smoking during pregnancy and its effects on the fetus. J Obstet Gynaecol Brit Commonwealth 1972;79:782–787.

3 Dalhamn T, Edfors M, Rylander R: Retention of cigarette smoke components in human lungs. Arch Environ Health 1968;17:746–748.

4 Coburn RF, Blakemore WS, Forster RE: Endogenous carbon monoxide production in man. J Clin Invest 1963;42:1172–1178.

5 Schmid R: Hyperbilirubinemia; in Stanbury JB, Wyngaarden JB, Fredrickson DS (eds): The Metabolic Basis of Inherited Disease. New York, McGraw-Hill, 1972, pp 1141–1178.

6 Ayres SM, Mueller HS, Gregory JJ, Giannelli S, Penny JL: Systemic and myocardial hemodynamic responses to relatively small concentrations of carboxyhemoglobin (COHB). Arch Environ Health 1969;18:699–709.

7 Adams JD, Erickson HH, Stone HL: The effects of carbon monoxide on coronary hemodynamics and left ventricular function in the conscious dog; in: Proc 1st Annu Conf on Evironmental Toxicology. Aerospace Medical Research Laboratory, 1970, TR-70-102, pp 107–124.

8 Cohen SI, Deane M, Goldsmith JR: Carbon monoxide and survival from myocardial infarction. Arch Environ Health 1969;19:510–517.

9 Ayres SM, Giannelli S, Mueller H: Myocardial and systemic responses to carboxy-hemoglobin. Ann NY Acad Sci 1970;174:268–293.

10 Anderson EW, Andelrnan RJ, Strauch JM, Fortuin NJ, Knelson JH: Effect of low-level carbon monoxide exposure on onset and duration of angina pectoris. Ann Intern Med 1973;79:46–50.

11 Allred EN, Bleecker ER, Chaitman BR, Dahms TE, Gottlieb SO, Hackney J, Pagano M, Sylvester RH, Walden SM, Warren J: Short-term effects of carbon monoxide on the exercise performance of subjects with coronary artery disease. N Engl J Med 1989; 321:1426–1432.

12 Calverley PMA, Leggett RJE, Flenley DC: Carbon monoxide and exercise tolerance in chronic bronchitis and emphysema. BMJ 1981;283:878–880.

13 Aronow WS: Smoking, carbon monoxide, and coronary heart disease. Circulation 1973;48:1169–1172.
14 Wald N, Howard S, Smith PG, Kjeldsen K: Association between atherosclerotic diseases and carboxyhaemoglobin levels in tobaco smokers. BMJ 1973;1:761–765.
15 Kjeldsen K, Damgaard F: Influence of prolonged carbon monoxide exposure and altitude hypoxia on serum lipids in man. Scand J Clin Lab Invest 1968;22(suppl 103): 16–19.
16 Astrup P, Kjeldsen K, Wanstrup J: Enhancing influence of carbon monoxide on the development of atheromatosis in cholesterol-fed rabbits. J Atheroscler Res 1967;7:343–354.
17 Wanstrup J, Kjeldsen K, Astrup P: Acceleration of spontaneous intimal-subintimal changes in rabbit aorta by a prolonged moderate carbon monoxide exposure. Acta Pathol Microbiol Scand 1969;75:353–362.
18 Webster WS, Clarkson TB, Lofland HB: Carbon monoxide-aggravated atherosclerosis in the squirrel monkey. Exp Mol Pathol 1970;13:36–50.
19 Malinow MR, McLaughlin P, Dhindsa DS, Metcalfe J, Ochsner AJ, Hill J, McNulty WP: Failure of carbon monoxide to induce myocardial infarction in cholesterol-fed cynomolgus monkeys *(Macaca fascicularis)*. Cardiovasc Res 1976;10:101–108.
20 Armitage AK, Davies RF, Turner DM: The effects of carbon monoxide on the development of atherosclerosis in the White Carneau pigeon. Atherosclerosis 1976;23: 333–344.
21 Kjeldsen K, Astrup P, Wanstrup J: Reversal of rabbit atheromatosis by hyperoxia. J Atheroscler Res 1969;10:173–178.
22 Kjeldsen K, Astrup P, Wanstrup J: Ultrastructural changes in the rabbit aorta after a moderate carbon monoxide exposure. Atherosclerosis 1972;16:67–82.
23 Hugod C, Hawkins LH, Kjeldsen K, Thomsen HK, Astrup P: Effect of carbon monoxide exposure on aortic and coronary intimal morphology in the rabbit. A re-evaluation. Atherosclerosis 1978;30:333–342.
24 Astrup P, Kjeldsen K: Model studies linking carbon monoxide and/or nicotine to arteriosclerosis and cardiovascular disease. Prev Med 1979;8:295–302.
25 Pfrender RE: Chronic carbon monoxide poisoning: A critical résumé. Ind Med Surg 1962;31:99–103.
26 Eckardt RE, MacFarland UN, Alarie YCE, Busey WM: The biologic effect from long-term exposure of primates to carbon monoxide. Arch Environ Health 1972; 25:381–387.
27 Jones RA, Strickland JA, Stunkard JA, Siegel J: Effects on experimental animals of long-term inhalation exposure to carbon monoxide. Toxicol Appl Pharmacol 1971; 19:46–53.
28 Kjeldsen K: Smoking and Atherosclerosis. Copenhagen, Munksgaard, 1969, pp 1–145.
29 Birnstingl MA, Brinson K, Chakrabarti BK: The effect of short-term exposure to carbon monoxide on platelet stickiness. Br J Surg 1971;58:837–839.
30 Russell MAH, Cole PV, Brown E: Absorption by non-smokers of carbon monoxide from room air polluted by tobacco smoke. Lancet 1973;i:576–579.
31 Srch M: Über die Bedeutung des Kohlenoxyds beim Zigarettenrauchen im Personenraftwageninneren. Dtsch Z Gesamte Gerichtl Med 1967;60:80–89.
32 Harke HP: Zum Problem des 'Passiv-Rauchens'. Münch Med Wochenschr 1970;112:2328–2334.
33 Editorial: Carbon monoxide, an old enemy forgot. Lancet 1981;ii:75–76.
34 Lawther PJ, Commins BT: Cigarette smoking and exposure to carbon monoxide. Ann NY Acad Sci 1970;174:135–147.

35 Godin G, Wright G, Shephard RJ: Urban exposure to carbon monoxide. Arch Environ Health 1972;25:305–313.
36 Ramsey JM: Estimating recent carbon monoxide exposures. Arch Environ Health 1962;5:308–318.
37 Moureu H: Carbon monoxide as a test for air pollution in Paris due to motor vehicle traffic. Proc R Soc Med 1964;57:1015–1020.
38 Curphey TJ, Hood LPL, Perkens NM: Carboxyhemoglobin in relation to air pollution and smoking: Post-mortem studies. Arch Environ Health 1965;10:179–185.
39 Cohen SI, Dorion G, Goldsmith JR, Permutt S: Carbon monoxide uptake by inspectors at a United States-Mexico border station. Arch Environ Health 1971;22:47–54.
40 Goldsmith JR, Terzaghi J, Hackney JD: Evaluation of fluctuating carbon monoxide exposures. Arch Environ Health 1963;7:647–663.
41 Haagen-Smit AJ: Carbon monoxide levels in city driving. Arch Environ Health 1966;12:548–551.

Dr. F.J.C. Roe, 19 Marryat Road, Wimbledon Common, London SW19 5BB (UK)

Weetman DF, Wood D (eds): Risk Factors for Cardiovascular Disease in Non-Smokers. Int. Workshop, Washington, Tyne and Wear, 1991. Basel, Karger, 1993, pp 129–136

# Environmental Tobacco Smoke

*Donald F. Weetman*

School of Health Sciences, University of Sunderland, UK

## *What Is Environmental Tobacco Smoke?*

Environmental tobacco smoke (ETS) is formed from burnt tobacco, part from the exhaled mainstream smoke (MS) and the rest from the sidestream smoke (SS) as a cigarette smoulders in an ashtray. There are many chemicals in ETS, but the composition of the mixture differs from other burnt organic material only with respect to the presence of the tobacco-specific alkaloid, nicotine.

There are subtle differences between SS and MS, arising mainly from the difference in the temperature of burning. Most of the ETS comes from SS, but only after it has aged and been diluted. The main differences between MS and ETS are indicated in table 1. It is not logical to consider exposure to ETS as equivalent to low dose smoking, so any arguments about the adverse health effects of ETS have to be made by establishing such an effect. The usual approach is through epidemiological studies.

## *Study Design*

There is no objective measure of chronic exposure to ETS, so a surrogate of exposure has been used in the various studies. In most cases, a non-smoker married to a smoker is considered to be exposed to ETS in the home: so a disease rate (events/possible events) can be measured for this group. A similar computation can be made in a non-smoking home, so the relative risk (RR) of exposure to ETS can be obtained by dividing the 'exposed' rate by the 'unexposed' rate. If the RR = 1 there is no effect of exposure of a non-smoker to ETS from the smoking of the spouse in the home (fig. 1).

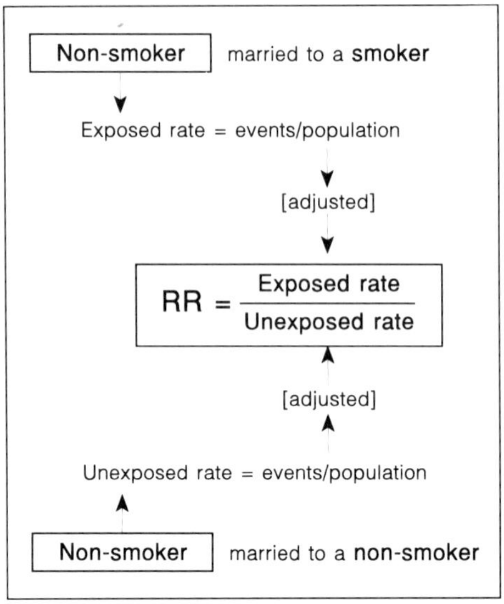


*Fig. 1.* Study design of effect of exposure of a non-smoker to ETS from the smoking of the spouse.

*Table 1.* Tobacco smoke from different sources

| Characteristic | MS | SS | ETS |
|---|---|---|---|
| Burning time | 2 s/min | 58 s/min | |
| Temperature of burning | 800 °C | 600 °C | |
| Particle size | large | small | small |
| pH | acid | alkaline | not measurable |
| Nicotine | particulate | gas | gas |
| NOx | NO | | $NO_2$ |
| Route of absorption | via mouth | | via nose |

MS = Mainstream smoke (i.e. that taken in by a smoker); SS = sidestream smoke (i.e. that emanating from a cigarette in an ashtray); ETS = environmental tobacco smoke. ETS is made up from exhaled MS and SS, but differs because it is both aged and diluted.

This general design can be used in either case-control (retrospective) or cohort (prospective) studies [see Lee, pp. 72–85]. In prospective studies, it is sometimes necessary to adjust the value for the disease rates to allow for differences in the populations compared, or between the cohort and the population at large. Such corrections are not needed in properly conducted case-control studies, because each case should be matched to one (or more) subject(s) with the control disease and other relevant characteristics (such as age, socio-economic status, education, income, occupation, housing and whatever else appears likely to confound the investigation).

The ingenious technique described above is intended to allow us to determine the effect of spousal smoking on the rate of disease. However, there are distinct problems in the accuracy of such estimates of exposure to ETS. No account is taken of exposure at work, in recreation, or to smoke in the home other than from the spouse. There is scope for the accuracy to be further compromised by misclassification of smokers and ex-smokers as non-smokers, especially as the smoking status (and thus the surrogate exposure) is determined by the response in questionnaires. It is possible to measure markers for exposure to tobacco smoke in either smokers or those exposed to ETS, but this is not done routinely, except in the most careful studies.

### *The Studies*

Twelve studies have been identified in the literature. I shall only consider those that have been subjected to the process of peer review (i.e. those that have been checked by an independent specialist at the editorial stage): the studies excluded at this stage are listed in table 2 [1, 2].

The acceptable studies are listed in table 3 [3–11]. Perhaps surprisingly, neither of the case-control studies [9, 10] yielded a statistically significant effect: it is usually easier to obtain a positive answer from this design than from cohort studies, although this simplicity sometimes leads to false identification of a risk factor for a disease (see Vandenbroucke and Pardoel [12], where, before the isolation of the virus, use of amyl nitrate was shown to be correlated with what we now call AIDS, with a high value for the relative risk, RR = 8.6).

There are four cohort studies that contained at least one statistically significant positive association between surrogate ETS exposure and cardiovascular disease. It is notable in this type of investigation that many tests for statistical significance are made: from all these comparisons, there are 14 significant effects from 115 tests (one would expect 6 if there were no effect with this number of comparisons and this level of statistical significance).

Of what quality are the studies that gave significant effects? Table 4 lists several factors that could have been measured, and would be expected to confound the investigation if not controlled for. In the studies by Helsing et al. [4] and Hirayama [6, 7], it is remarkable that so many potential confounders are ignored. Perhaps it is not surprising that the

*Table 2.* Five studies not considered

| Author | Events | RR | Reason for exclusion |
|---|---|---|---|
| Martin, 1986 | 23 | 2.4* | quoted but not published |
| He et al., 1989 [1] | 34 | 1.5* | in Chinese |
| Butler, 1990 [2] | 64 | 1.4 | abstract only |
| Palmer (?) | ? | 1.2 | unpublished |

* = Claimed to be statistically significant $p < 0.05$.

*Table 3.* ETS – CVD: epidemiology

| Design | Study | Disease | Events/possible | | Comparisons $p < 0.05$/total |
|---|---|---|---|---|---|
| | | | control | exposed | |
| Prospective | Garland, 1985 [3] | IHD | 2/203 | 17/492 | 0/10 |
| Prospective | Helsing et al., 1988 [4] | arterioscl HD | 677 | 1337 | 10/22[1] |
| Prospective | Svendsen et al., 1987 [11] | CHD | 8/959 | 5/286 | 2/17[1] |
| Prospective | Gillis et al., 1984 [5] | IHD | 30/489 | 54/1,295 | 1/5[1] |
| Prospective | Hirayama, 1981 [6] | IHD | total 406 | | 0/4 |
| Prospective | Hirayama, 1984 [7] | IHD | 118/21,859 | 376/69,645 | 1/3[1] |
| C–C | Lee et al., 1986 [10] | IHD + stroke | 200 | 200 | 0/30 |
| C–C | Humble et al., 1990 [9] | all CVD | total 76 | | 0/24 |

[1] Consider these four positive studies in detail.

*Table 4.* Missing evidence (potential confounders) in the significant studies

| Factor | Hirayama [6, 7] | Helsing et al. [4] | Svendsen et al. [11][1] | Gillis et al. [5][2] |
|---|---|---|---|---|
| Smoke marker | missing | missing | present | missing |
| Menopausal status | missing | missing | men only | missing |
| Family history of CVD | missing | missing | missing | missing |
| BP data | missing | missing | present | present |
| Body weight/mass | missing | missing | present | present |
| High fat diet | missing | missing | plasma chol. | plasma chol. |
| Alcohol consumption | present | missing | present | missing |
| Diabetes | missing | missing | missing | missing |
| Exercise | missing | missing | missing | missing |

[1] Svendsen et al. used top 15% males at CVD risk.
[2] Cohort of Gillis et al. too small (PS was 89% AS).

Helsing et al. study gave 10 of the 14 significant associations between surrogate exposure to ETS and cardiovascular deaths, because it is the least controlled of all the positive studies. When one looks at the methodology, the study consists of linking death certificate information with a census report of several factors obtained 12 years earlier in Washington County, Maryland. Amongst these factors was self-professed smoking status; however, this question was asked only once in 1963. Any non-smokers taking up the habit after 1963, and any smokers misclassified as non-smokers in the census, would result in any effects of cigarette smoking being attributed to ETS exposure. This study also failed to trace a high proportion of the original cohort (2.3%/year as far as can be determined from the paper), because it recorded deaths in Washington County only. Who could tell what effect on the result would have occurred if the missing persons had been traced and added to the study? One is tempted to conclude that this study has been published because of the political importance of the result, rather than because of its quality.

The Hirayama cohort study has had great impact on public health policies. The original aim of the study was to examine the effects of life-style factors on mortality in Japan, especially to determine if consumption of green-yellow vegetables could reduce cancer incidence. However, it was from this study that the first claim appeared that spousal exposure to ETS was associated with lung cancer in non-smokers [6].

A total of 265,118 adults over 40 years of age were recruited to the study from 29 health centres in 6 prefectures in 1965. Information about the life-style of each subject was obtained at the outset from a one-page questionnaire [reproduced in 13]. A second single-page questionnaire, this time filled in by a public health nurse in a standardized interview, was administered to a randomly selected 3% sample in 1971. The cause of death was taken from death certificates. In 1981, Hirayama [6] reported that spousal exposure to ETS was not associated with an increased incidence of cardiovascular disease ($RR = 1.03$, $p = 0.393$); however, 3 years later, a significant effect was found ($RR = 1.31$, $p = 0.0191$; table 3).

There are faults in the Hirayama study. The cohort was assembled for convenience, rather than as a random sample, which resulted in information being obtained from an unbalanced population. Reference to the United Nations Demographic Yearbook of 1976 shows that old people (over 70) are 7-fold underrepresented, and that farm workers are 4-fold overrepresented in the cohort. The reliance on death certificates for the cause of death is unreliable [14]. Some of the putative risk factors for cardiovascular diseases not considered by Hirayama are contained in table 4, and emphasizes the problem intrinsic to the identification of risk factors in the course of a cohort study set up for other purposes: the important, potentially confounding information is not collected because this was not the purpose of the study.

The standard of the two remaining studies is much higher than those of Helsing and Hirayama. Unfortunately, there are still important possible confounders not controlled for in these studies. The study of Gillis et al. [5, 8] takes no account of a family history of cardiovascular disease, diabetes, menopausal status, etc. (table 4). The small size of the study also represents a problem. As the reported effect of spousal exposure to ETS was almost 90% of that of smoking, one wonders if the authors have been unfortunate in selecting an atypical population (for ischaemic heart disease, smokers RR = 2.27; surrogate exposure to ETS RR = 2.01, 95% confidence limits = 1.21–3.35). If this result were typical, it would not be possible to demonstrate any effect of cigarette smoking!

The study of Svendsen et al. [11] considers a subpopulation of the Multiple Risk Factor Intervention Trial (MRFIT). There was a significant effect for death from any cause for non-smoking men living with a smoking wife (adjusted RR = 1.79, 95% confidence limits 1.17–2.76), but neither fatal nor non-fatal coronary heart disease events showed a significant effect ($p > 0.05$). Entry to this trial was restricted to the 15% of men considered to be most at risk from cardiovascular disease, as determined in the Framingham study. Thus the subjects possessed two of the three risk factors thought to be most important with respect to cardiovascular disease: cigarette smoking, high blood cholesterol levels, or being classified as hypertensive. As the effects of spousal smoking in non-smokers was determined, all the subjects must have been hypertensive and have had high blood cholesterol levels. This highly selected study population cannot provide useful information about the risks of normal individuals to ETS.

However, the Svendsen study does show that it is possible to conduct a controlled epidemiological study of the effects of ETS by the spousal smoking status design. This exemplary study was so much more carefully performed than the others described in this paper (table 4). A marker for smoking status was measured, and the end point was determined by a panel of cardiologists who were unaware of the treatment, or in this case subgroup, of the deceased. Any future studies need to be designed with at least the care and attention to detail found in the Svendsen study.

## *Conclusion*

It is not possible to conclude that a risk to cardiovascular health has been established from the epidemiological studies considered in this paper.

Each of the studies is flawed in at least one major way. If there are to be more studies, and the importance of cardiovascular diseases suggests there should be, one can only hope that they will be conducted in a careful and objective way. At the present time, this author agrees with this aspect of Spitzer et al. [15]: 'After an initial review of the literature, we determined that insufficient studies of high quality had been done in the area of cardiovascular disease to warrant comment in our review at the present time.' It is against this background that one should view the claims in the media, based on purportedly balanced scientific publications [e.g. see 16], that ETS is responsible for 37,000 deaths from cardiovascular disease each year in the USA. Perhaps these journalists, and the authors who provide their scientific sources, should read Feinstein [17], who berates the low scientific standards that can be found in much epidemiology.

## *References*


1 He Y, Li L, Wan Z, Li L, Zheng X, Jia G: Passive smoking and coronary heart disease in women. China J Prev Med 1989;23:19–22.

2 Butler T: The relationship of passive smoking to various health outcomes among Seventh-Day Adventists in California (abstract). VIIth World Conference on Tobacco and Health 1990;316:2.

3 Garland C, Barrett-Connor E, Suarez L, Criqui MH, Wingard DL: Effects of passive smoking on ischemic heart disease mortality of nonsmokers: a prospective study. Am J Epidemiol 1985;121:645–650.

4 Helsing KJ, Sandler DP, Comstock GW, Chee E: Heart disease mortality in nonsmokers living with smokers. Am J Epidemiol 1988;127:915–922.

5 Gillis CR, Hole DJ, Hawthorne VM, Boyle P: The effect of environmental tobacco smoke in two urban communities in the west of Scotland. Eur J Respir Dis 1984;65 (suppl 133):121–126.

6 Hirayama T: Non-smoking wives of heavy smokers have higher risk of lung cancer: A study from Japan. Br Med J 1981;282:183–185.

7 Hirayama T: Lung cancer in Japan: Effects of nutrition and passive smoking; in Mizell M, Correa P (eds): Lung Cancer: Causes and Prevention. New York, Verlag Chemie International, 1984, pp 175–195.

8 Hole DJ, Gillis CR, Chopra C, Hawthorne VM: Passive smoking and cardiorespiratory health in a general population in the west of Scotland. Br Med J 1989;299:423–427.

9 Humble C, Croft J, Gerber A, Casper M, Hames CG, Tyroler HA: Passive smoking and 20-year cardiovascular disease mortality among nonsmoking wives, Evans County, Georgia. Am J Public Health 1990;80:599–601.

10 Lee P, Chamberlain J, Alderson M: Relationship of passive smoking to risk of lung cancer and other smoking associated diseases. Br J Cancer 1986;54:97–105.

11 Svendsen KH, Kuller LH, Martin MJ, Ockene JH: Effects of passive smoking in the multiple risk factor intervention trial. Am J Epidemiol 1987;126:783–795.

12 Vandenbroucke JP, Pardoel VPAM: An autopsy of epidemiologic methods: The case of 'poppers' in the early epidemic of the acquired immunodeficiency syndrome (AIDS). Am J Epidemiol 1989;129:455–457.

13 Hirayama T: Life-Style and Mortality. A Large-Scale Census-Based Cohort Study in Japan. Basel, Karger, 1990.
14 Hill AB: A Short Textbook of Medical Statistics, ed 11. London, Arnold, 1984.
15 Spitzer WO, Lawrence V, Dales R, Hill G, Archer MC, Clark P, Abenhaim L, Hardy J, Sampalis J, Pinfold SP, Morgan PP: Links between passive smoking and disease: A best-evidence synthesis. A report of the working group on passive smoking. Clin Invest Med 1990;13:17–42.
16 Glantz SA, Parmley WW: Passive smoking and heart disease: Epidemiology, physiology and biochemistry. Circulation 1991;83:1–12.
17 Feinstein AR: Scientific standards in epidemiologic studies of the menace of daily life. Science 1988;242:1257–1263.

Prof. Donald F. Weetman, School of Health Sciences, University of Sunderland, Sunderland SR1 3SD (UK)

Weetman DF, Wood D (eds): Risk Factors for Cardiovascular Disease in Non-Smokers. Int. Workshop, Washington, Tyne and Wear, 1991. Basel, Karger, 1993, pp 137–141

# The Multifactorial Aetiology of Coronary Heart Disease: A Dangerous Delusion

*James McCormick*

Department of Community Health, Trinity College, Dublin, Ireland

To date, something over 300 'risk markers' have been described for coronary heart disease (CHD). I use the term 'risk marker' advisedly, because although every epidemiologist recognizes that a risk factor is a factor that is associated with an altered probability of disease, and that risk factors are not necessarily causally related, the language of those who talk about risk factors often imputes, sometimes unwittingly, causal relationships.

The list of risk markers now includes cigarette smoking, serum cholesterol, high blood pressure, obesity, diabetes, low levels of high density lipoproteins, high levels of low density lipoproteins, thiazide diuretics, not drinking, not exercising, not having siestas, not eating fish especially mackerel, living in Scotland, speaking English as a mother tongue, having a high level of phobic anxiety, being scrupulous about keeping appointments, not taking cod liver oil and snoring. Recently baldness has been added to the list. This may be associated with increased androgen production, so the good news is that your sex life may be better; the bad news is that you will probably die while making love. The important associations include age, being male, a family history and being poor.

These apparent riches are dross: the number of 'risk markers' is a monument to industry, but a reflection of ignorance. The prevalent notion that saying that a disease has a multifactorial etiology is useful, is a dangerous delusion. All diseases, and indeed everything that happens to us, is the end result of the interplay of many factors. The only necessary cause of my being here today is the accidental conjunction of a particular sperm and ovum some years ago! Nonetheless, that happy union, although necessary, is not a sufficient cause of my presence.

The term 'multifactorial' when applied to disease aetiology is a tautology that has led to unreal expectations and delusion. Nobody refers to pneumococcal pneumonia as having a multifactorial aetiology, although previous experience in pneumococci, smoking, nutrition and immunocompetence, may all determine the occurrence of disease. Those diseases whose causes are known, infectious and parasitic diseases, vitamin deficiencies, some endocrine disorders, can all be treated satisfactorily and some can be prevented. Diseases whose cause is unknown are seldom satisfactorily treatable and none is preventable. Multifactorial is a synonym for 'unknown', and is thus a euphemism for ignorance.

I think chronic disease epidemiology has reached the end of a road. It will never give us aetiological answers about chronic diseases. The best it can do is to suggest hypotheses which can then be pursued in the molecular biological field. The approach of epidemiology has been incredibly simplistic, where everything that we really understand turns out to be incredibly complex. Blood clotting is much more than the transfer of fibrinogen to fibrin; we now understand something about it. We are beginning as we heard today, very excitingly, to understand a little bit about lipid metabolism, and I believe the future of coronary heart disease understanding is in fact not going to stem from further epidemiological studies, particularly of the case-control design, but will come from laboratory studies.

The dangerous delusion to which I referred is that a knowledge of risk markers provides a strategy for prevention, when the cause of the disease is unknown. Most of the risk markers which have been described have an uncertain or non-existent causal role, yet the ascription of aetiological significance brings in its wake unreal expectations of prevention. Causal relationships should be susceptible to experimental proof: that is, an experiment which alters the risk marker should result in an altered instance of disease. And the critical experiment in medicine, as Peter Lee has pointed out to us earlier today, is the randomized control trial.

Table 1 summarizes the results of a meta-analysis of such studies carried out by Petr Skrabenek and myself [1]. Almost all the studies to date have been carried out in middle-aged men, in whom the risk of CHD, while still small, is greater than in women.

Table 2 summarizes cholesterol intervention trials. The results show that when you consider CHD deaths there is a gain of 8 deaths in 115,176 man-years, but for total deaths there was a loss of 35.

Further evidence of ignorance stems from the conflicting nature of advice which derives from inadequate information and lack of secure

*Table 1.* Multiple risk factor intervention trials (828,000 man-years)

| CHD deaths | | Total deaths | |
|---|---|---|---|
| intervention | control | intervention | control |
| 1,015 | 1,049 | 2,909 | 2,947 |

Data from WHO, Göteborg, MRFIT, Helsinki/Oslo [cf. 1].

*Table 2.* Cholesterol drug intervention trials (115,176 man-years)

| CHD deaths | | Total deaths | |
|---|---|---|---|
| intervention | control | intervention | control |
| 92 | 100 | 275 | 240 |

Data from WHO, LRC-CPPT, Helsinki [cf. 1].

knowledge. Most of you will be aware from reading your daily newspapers that butter, milk and cream, which were bad, may now be good. Alcohol, short of drunkenness and gross excess, is almost certainly good for your coronary arteries, but has yet to become the centre-piece of 'Heartwatch' or other similar programmes of public education, which should perhaps be better described as 'public exhortation'.

CHD has been described as 'the greatest epidemic of modern times'; at least until the emergence of AIDS. In fact, it is not a new disease; James Mackenzie, when he was a general practitioner in Burnley at the turn of the century, saw a great deal of it [2]. It is, nonetheless, an important disease, and is the commonest single disgnosis to be recorded on death certificates. However, the median age of death for men who are certified as dying from this cause is about 75; and for women the median age of death is somewhat older.

People tend to talk as if coronary artery disease was a single entity, whereas the clinical manifestations may represent the end point of different pathological processes. Myocardial infarction in a relatively young man, that entity which reasonably used to be called 'coronary thrombosis', may indeed be primarily a clotting phenomenon, different from stable angina in a 68-year-old woman or infarction in an 80-year-old. Young men's 'coronaries' are associated with smoking (although smoking is not a necessary cause), an association which disappears with advancing age [3].

Health promotionists are now implying that dying of a coronary is the wages of sin, the result of smoking, eating unsuitable food, adding salt, preferring to be a couch potato rather than a jogger, and that eschewing such noxious habits is the path of virtuous living. The reality is that the most we can hope for is that death may be postponed, and it is certainly not preventable, and as Petr Skrabanek has reminded us, life itself is a universally fatal, sexually transmitted disease.

Not dying of CHD ensures the possibility of an alternative mode of death. Not all the alternatives are immediately attractive. Those of us who work in clinical practice cannot fail to be aware of the increasing numbers of people who are living to die the slow death of senescence.

Much of our striving for health seems to be a cause of unhappiness and iatrogenic harm. For most doctors, health is the absence of disease, which has led at least one wag to describe the healthy as the inadequately investigated; for most people health is feeling good; for the World Health Organization health is a state of complete physical, mental and social well-being, a state which according to the late Henry Miller, the distinguished Dean of Medicine at Newcastle University, was only achievable in acute mania and at the moment of orgasm. Myers [4] assembled the composite picture of an individual with a low risk of CHD and presumably particularly healthy, as 'an effeminate municipal worker or embalmer, completely lacking in physical or mental alertness, and without drive, ambition or competitive spirit; who has never attempted to meet a deadline of any kind; a man with poor appetite subsisting on fruit and vegetables laced with corn and whale oil, detesting tobacco, spurning ownership of radio, television or motorcar, with full head of hair but scrawny and unathletic appearance, yet constantly straining his puny muscles by exercise. Low in income, blood pressure, uric acid and cholesterol, he has taken nicotinic acid, pyridoxine and long-term anticoagulant therapy ever since his prophylactic castration'.

In the knowledge that for the most part our longevity is encoded in our genes, it seems to me that health is coping with the slings and arrows of outrageous fortune, rather than a vain search for the elixir of life. This definition allows health for the handicapped, the disabled and the old, and even allows the possibility of dying healthy. Preconditions of health are a sufficiency of money to provide food, clothing and shelter, and above all, being loved. In these circumstances, we should be encouraged to live lives of modified hedonism, so that we may enjoy to the full the only life that we are ever likely to have.

## *References*


1 McCormick JS, Skrabanek P: Coronary heart disease is not preventable by population interventions. Lancet 1988;ii:839–841.

2 McCormick JS: James Mackenzie and coronary heart disease. JR Coll Gen Pract 1981;31;26–30.

3 Seltzer CC: Framingham study data and 'established wisdom' about cigarette smoking and coronary heart disease. J Clin Epidemiol 1989;42:743–750.

4 Myers GS, quoted by Zola IK: Medicine as an institution of social control; in Cox C, Mead A (eds): A Sociology of Medical Practice. London, Collier-Macmillan, 1975, pp 170–185.


James McCormick, Department of Community Health, Trinity College, Dublin (Ireland)

# Overall Findings

Weetman DF, Wood D (eds): Risk Factors for Cardiovascular Disease in Non-Smokers. Int. Workshop, Washington, Tyne and Wear, 1991. Basel, Karger, 1993, pp 142–146

## Conclusion of the Workshop

*Donald F. Weetman*

School of Health Sciences, University of Sunderland, UK

At the end of a very long, informative and rewarding day, it is worthwhile to attempt to review the findings. Perhaps, too, it is worthwhile emphasizing why the workshop chose to look at non-smokers. To cover the problem in one day, as was essential from an organizational point of view, it was decided to avoid the much considered topic of cigarette smoking and cardiovascular disease. There is a vast amount of information available elsewhere on this topic [see e.g. 1, 2]. Further, cigarette smokers are in a minority in most western countries (generally between 20 and 40% of adults smoke [3]), so it was thought worthwhile looking at the problems of the majority.

In the absence of persuasive evidence to the contrary, most instances of non-traumatic sudden death are attributed to cardiovascular disease, most frequently coronary thrombosis. In the Framingham study (26-year follow-up), sudden death was responsible for 50% of the male and 39% of the female cardiovascular deaths [4]. Ventricular fibrillation may be the means of sudden death, but what initiates the fibrillation? A previous infarction of the myocardium is undoubtedly important, but so too are reflexes, perhaps particularly so in the proportion of deaths where the lesions to the myocardium and coronary arteries are not extensive.

Two categories of risk for cardiovascular disease were apparent from this workshop. First, there is immutable risk, which is represented by a genetic component detectable in families, perhaps a predisposition to diabetes, the way we handle dietary fat, etc. For all of these factors, the die is cast at birth, so we have to accept our fate; nothing can be done to reduce the risk.

Although of a smaller size, environmental risks are more important, because we *can* act to minimize these. Not all activities or individual characteristics considered in this workshop were equally disadvantageous. Impaired respiratory function predicts a poor prognosis for cardiovascular disease. A useful distinction was drawn between sport and exercise: some activity that involves physical effort is recommended, especially if the participant derives pleasure from it. Perhaps the good news is that there is no strong evidence that associates exposure to lead, carbon monoxide, and ETS with cardiovascular disease in non-smokers.

Many of the risks that have been identified depend upon evidence from epidemiological studies [5]; now there are thought to be more than 300 according to Prof. McCormick, some of which are bizarre in the extreme. There was a fundamental difference in the way these were viewed by the different presenters. The pertinent question is: Should they be considered to be 'risk factors', or would it be more accurate to describe them as 'risk markers'? The implications behind the choice of words to describe them are diametrically opposed. If we choose to use 'risk factors', the implication is that the influence can be reduced or even avoided; whereas, the use of 'marker' suggests a loose association of two life events, just connecting the influence (marker) with the outcome (disease or cause of death), with no casuality implied.

From a health education perspective, it is essential to consider the influences to be 'factors', so the consequent 'good advice' is to avoid the influence, if at all possible. As we are exhorted repeatedly from the media, do not eat animal fat; do not smoke cigarettes; get your hypertension under control; avoid stress; only consume moderate amounts of alcohol; eat more fibre; do not avoid exercise, and so on. Health programmes to induce such changes in behaviour now constitute a major endeavour in the western world. A veritable industry of persuasion has grown up.

One wonders about the wisdom of such advice. How many children are persuaded to become vegetarians because of the advice received from well-meaning, but poorly aware, school teachers? If the simplistic message is wrong, then changes in behaviour will be irrelevant to health. As we have seen today, the more one looks at the detail, the less we really know.

The very few lives saved from cardiovascular death by the massive intervention programmes, as highlighted by Prof. McCormick, are worth pondering. If one considers death from 'all causes', there are in fact no lives saved in the reported trials, so it seems that such health intervention programmes are nonsensical. Perhaps the morbidity of the participants improved, but if so, one has to remember the subjectivity involved in reaching this conclusion.

Without an overall benefit in the form of saved lives, why do we persist in offering what appears to be irrelevant advice? The answer may lie in the existence of the health education programmes. Once you have charged somebody with a task, it is very difficult to fault him or her from performing it diligently. Perhaps, too, it is difficult to admit the paucity of our underlying knowledge, and that we do not know how to reduce the death toll. Selectivity of evidence enters the consideration. The reduced cardiovascular mortality in the North Karelia Risk Factor Reduction Initiative is claimed to be a successful programme, whilst the comparable reduction in adjoining Kuopio, and all other areas of Finland for that matter, where there was no such programme, receives no emphasis [6]. It is quite clear that we have not yet identified all the influences. There is much we do not understand. More research into identification of these factors is needed before we can contemplate embarking on effective intervention programmes.

One cannot help suspecting that changing the behaviour of people becomes an end in itself, whereas it should be a means to an end. If one accepts the case described above, the fundamental error does not reside in the programme, but in the decision to set up the programme. If the vox populi is that 'they should do something about it', one can start to understand why politicians provide funds for this very visible activity before next facing the electorate.

The other way at looking at the problem of reducing cardiovascular mortality is represented by the school of thought that argues that we must do something. This too is flawed. It is the same pseudo-scientific approach that is prevalent in the attitude of some to some environmental hazards [7]. The argument maintains that we cannot afford to wait until the problem is resolved scientifically before we act. Although this may seem to be a sensible approach because there is no disadvantage in it, this is not the case. Any action involves costs, so with the limited funds available, it may well be that the money could be used more prudently elsewhere. Well-intended purposes are not sufficient grounds to rush into initiatives that will fail ultimately.

By some strange reasoning, some members of western society seem to have accepted the nostrum that serious disease is in principle preventable. Such belief has to be considered in the context of the small improvements in adult life expectancy in recent times [8], so presumably any gain on one front has to be offset against a more or less comparable loss elsewhere. Equally, it is true that a few individual cases of serious diseases can be prevented; vide the evidence from occupational medicine and industrial hygiene, which indicates that a reduction in some occupational diseases can be achieved. However, it is not at all clear how the very special circumstances that apply in the workplace can be related to the population at large in their non-industrial setting. Even in occupational medicine, the overall gains are comparatively small, although, of course, they will be of immense benefit to the individual. If one considers cancer, a medical outcome which is probably surrounded by less uncertainty than cardiovascular disease, Doll and Peto [9] have estimated that only 4–8% is industrially derived. Furthermore, these figures relate to exposure in the past, and standards of industrial hygiene have since improved remarkably, so the potential for current gains would probably be much less.

Whatever has been said above is really a plea for the funding of more carefully controlled research into the possible causation and mechanisms of cardiovascular disease. One is not optimistic that a fundamentally new approach will come from epidemiology, which is particularly prone to generate false leads [10], so a fuller understanding of pathological mechanisms and better management of patients seem to offer the best prospects.

Cardiovascular diseases contribute the largest proportion of deaths today [8]. Even if we cannot all agree to think in terms of risk factors, because of the implied causality of this terminology, some characteristics, intrinsic or behavioural, seem to be more dangerous than others. Genetic constitution and being poor seem to be substantial and immutable influences. It seems likely that there may be differences in coronary artery disease in men and women, yet findings from the former are quite often incautiously applied to the latter [11]. Perhaps the most persuasive evidence from epidemiology comes from intervention studies, where a suspected factor is removed or reduced from a population and a reduction in disease incidence follows. However, in the Multiple Risk Factor Intervention Trial (MRFIT) there was a non-significant difference in the deaths from coronary heart disease between the intervention and control groups, even though the target reduction in cigarette smoking was exceeded in the intervention group [12, 13]. These paradoxical findings are usually glossed over by health educationalists [see e.g. 3 and many other papers in the same issue of this journal]. It has also been claimed that the Framingham findings run quite contrary to the consensus view of the Surgeon General, which appears to be the basis for most health education and intervention programmes aimed at cardiovascular diseases [14].

The points made above should not be interpreted as an attempt to dismiss out of hand the contributions of health education and interventions in reducing the impact of cardiovascular diseases. The results so far have been a disappointment. If the general population is promised too great a benefit, when the truth emerges, as it will eventually, the whole process will come to be held in low regard. Subsequent preventive medical programmes will then suffer. As with most difficulties of the sort considered here, the answer may lie in a better quality of education of the health educationist. This is what we seek to achieve on our courses at the University of Sunderland, so we must take every opportunity to get our students to think for themselves. Suppressing uncomfortable anomalies and inconsistencies in the evidence is no way of achieving this. There is also a clear need for more meetings between sceptical medical scientists and the health educators, so that those who deliver the advice to the public do not misstate their case.

## *References*


1 Anon: The Health Consequences of Smoking: Cardiovascular Disease. A Report of the Surgeon General. Washington, US Government Printing Office, 1989.
2 Diana JN: Tobacco Smoking and Atherosclerosis: Pathogenesis and Cellular Mechanisms. New York, Plenum Press, 1990.
3 Karvonen MJ: Health challenges of the developed world. Hygie 1992;11(suppl):18–23.
4 Lerner D, Kannel W: Patterns of coronary heart disease morbidity and mortality in the sexes: A 26-year follow-up of the Framingham population. Am Heart J 1986;111:383–390.
5 Hopkins PN, Williams RR: A survey of 246 suggested coronary risk factors. Atherosclerosis 1981;40:1–52.
6 Skrabanek P, McCormick J: Follies and Fallacies in Medicine. Glasgow, Tarragon Press, 1989, pp 21–58.
7 Efron E: The Apocalyptics. How Environmental Politics Controls What We Know about Cancer. New York, Simon & Schuster, 1984, pp 231–383.
8 Jacobson B, Smith A, Whitehead M: The Nation's Health. A Strategy for the 1990s, rev ed. London, King Edward's Hospital Fund for London, 1991, pp 22–29.
9 Doll R, Peto R: The causes of cancer: Quantitative estimates of avoidable risk in the United States today. J Natl Cancer Inst 1981;66:1191–1303.
10 Feinstein AR: Scientific standards in epidemiologic studies of the menace of daily life. Science 1988;242:1257–1263.
11 Eaker ED, Packard B, Wenger K, Clarkson TB, Tyroler HA: Coronary artery disease in women. Am J Cardiol 1988;61:641–644.
12 Stallones RA: Mortality and the Multiple Risk Factor Intervention Trial. Am J Epidemiol 1983;117:647–650.
13 Group MRFITR: Multiple Risk Factor Intervention Trial. Risk factor changes and mortality results. JAMA 1982;248:1465–1477.
14 Seltzer CC: Framingham study data and 'established wisdom' about cigarette smoking and coronary heart disease. J Clin Epidemiolol 1989;42:743–750.


Prof. Donald F. Weetman, School of Health Sciences,
University of Sunderland, Sunderland SR1 3SD (UK)

# Subject Index